Real People Need Real Food

Real People Need Real Food

A Guide to Healthy Eating for Families living in a Fast Food World

Laura Einbinder RD, LDN and
Kate Scarlata RD, LDN

iUniverse, Inc.
New York Lincoln Shanghai

Real People Need Real Food
A Guide to Healthy Eating for Families living in a Fast Food World

Copyright © 2008 by Laura Einbinder and Kate Scarlata

All rights reserved. No part of this book may be used or reproduced by any means, graphic, electronic, or mechanical, including photocopying, recording, taping or by any information storage retrieval system without the written permission of the publisher except in the case of brief quotations embodied in critical articles and reviews.

iUniverse books may be ordered through booksellers or by contacting:

iUniverse
2021 Pine Lake Road, Suite 100
Lincoln, NE 68512
www.iuniverse.com
1-800-Authors (1-800-288-4677)

Because of the dynamic nature of the Internet, any Web addresses or links contained in this book may have changed since publication and may no longer be valid.

You should not undertake any diet/exercise regimen recommended in this book before consulting your personal physician. Neither the author nor the publisher shall be responsible or liable for any loss or damage allegedly arising as a consequence of your use or application of any information or suggestions contained in this book.

ISBN: 978-0-595-46760-0 (pbk)
ISBN: 978-0-595-91054-0 (ebk)

Printed in the United States of America

Contents

Introduction vii

Chapter 1: Why Do We Feel Fat and Tired? 1
Chapter 2: Mindful Eating: Eating as if Your Life Depended on It! 10
Chapter 3: Kids Keeping Pace in a Fast-Food World 19
Chapter 4: Balancing the Plate: Serving Up Variety and Proportion 31
Chapter 5: Healthy Eating for All: A Look at the 2005 USDA Food Pyramid Guidelines 46
Chapter 6: Grocery Shopping Guidelines 62
Chapter 7: Eating on the Run: It's All in the Planning! 79
Chapter 8: Back to Basics: Eating Real Food 95
Chapter 9: Where's the Beef? Less Is More When It Comes to Meat 107
Chapter 10: Food Labels: How to Read One 117
Chapter 11: A Word about Exercise 124
Chapter 12: Vitamins, Minerals, Phytochemicals, and Functional Foods: Food for Thought 130
Chapter 13: Food Connections: From Field to Table 147

Reference List 149
Recommended Cookbooks 153
Recipes 157

BMI Chart for Adults..203
Bibliography...205

Introduction

"Happy is he who sits down to the dinner provided for him without thought of what he must leave out, with a mind free for social pleasure, secure in the skill and knowledge of his cook. Happier still are the children brought up under the watchful eye of another who understands the laws of health and holds them in high regard."
—Mary Swartz Rose, PhD, *Feeding the Family,* 1940

The pursuit of optimal health and wellness for both of us has been a journey of exploration and enlightenment. We have had our share of obstacles and challenges; none have been insurmountable, but they have changed the framework we use to measure our personal goals. Our experiences on this personal journey as mothers and wives, our combined decades of experience providing nutrition counseling to thousands of individuals, and our constant quest for the best nutrition information and research available, prompted us to write this book together.

What is good nutrition? The old yet profound adage "You are what you eat" is one that we honestly take to heart and fully believe. When you balance your diet by choosing healthy, chemical-free foods, not only will you feel more energetic and balanced, you will also lower your risk of illness.

We hope to **entertain and educate mainstream American families** on how to eat with joy and gusto without the need for intensive diets or fast food meals in the quick paced world in which we live. We encourage the reader to embrace personalized nutritional change—not by giving general recommendations, but by facilitating a journey of self discovery by offering specific steps to optimizing health and well being. This book **deciphers**

current scientific research with a humorous approach bound to have the reader reaching for something good to eat one moment, and laughing the next.

This book is designed with families in mind. It **brings the reader to a new awareness of** the many obstacles in American society that influence our eating habits. This **action oriented** book provides simple tips for **streamlining meal planning** from grocery shopping to meal preparation. It lists valuable references such as trusted websites, fantastic cookbooks, and a multitude of the authors' *tried and true,* **delicious healthy recipes.** Some of the many topics covered include: **deciphering food labels** for the everyday grocery shopper, providing **recommendations for nutritional supplements,** defining the difference **between mindless and mindful eating,** and thinking about **exercise as a pleasurable family activity** not a chore. We hope you will feel empowered to make and indulge in healthy changes leading to **better health for the body and the soul.**

Chapter 1:
Why Do We Feel Fat and Tired?

Be willing to be a beginner every single morning.
—Meister Eckhart

> Objectives:
> - Why are Americans gaining weight at an alarming rate?
> - Why are we more stressed and tired than ever before?
> - What can we do to inspire the change we want for ourselves, our families, and the world in which we live?

As a whole, Americans are getting fatter. The number of Americans who are overweight or obese has increased substantially over the past several decades. The latest National Health and Nutrition Examination Survey (NHANES) data indicate 65 percent of U.S. adults aged 20 years and older are overweight. In addition, 16 percent of children and adolescents ages 6–19 in the United States are overweight. *(http://www.cdc.gov/od/oc/media/pressrel/fs050419.htm)*

'Overweight' and 'obese' are both labels for ranges of weight that are greater than what is generally considered healthy for a given height. For adults, overweight and obesity ranges are determined by using weight and height to calculate a number called the "body mass index" (BMI). BMI is used because, for most people, it correlates with their amount of body fat.

- o An adult who has a BMI between 25 and 29.9 is considered overweight.

o   An adult who has a BMI of 30 or higher is considered obese.

See the **BMI Chart for Adults** to assess your own BMI at the end of this book.

Source: http://www.cdc.gov/nccdphp/dnpa/obesity/defining.htm

It is difficult to pinpoint a single reason for this alarming trend. Advances in technology, the increased consumption of fast food, and the trend toward more sedentary lifestyle choices are all likely factors. We live in an over stimulating world. Down time is almost nonexistent. Busy family schedules further complicate our pursuit of health. When can we actually prepare a home-cooked meal? Almost without realizing it, our lifestyles have spun out of control. Several common experiences described here contribute to this phenomenon.

Bulk Food and the Expanding Inventory

The experience of bulk-food shopping at one of our megastores—Costco, Sam's Club, Wal-Mart—is uniquely American: a celebration of "extreme" shopping at its greatest. What could be better than buying supersized, pre-packaged food at ridiculously low prices? We can bring home a year's supply of tuna fish or canned peaches packaged all in one can!

My grocery inventory had continued to grow as I took advantage of these "bargains." At first, just my kitchen cabinets and spare closets began to fill up with inventory. Then I had to make room in the garage, and I kept telling my husband that I needed to buy a spare freezer and refrigerator for all of the other food items I wanted to stock. Unfortunately, I had not found an effective inventory control system. I forgot that I had ten five-pound bags of flour in the upstairs hall closet or that there was another bag of potatoes on the workbench outside in the garage.

Sometimes after completing an extreme shopping trip, however, I found myself still shopping at the local grocery store in order to make something for dinner. And random thoughts began to seep into my subconscious: How long *will* it take a family of five to eat a gallon bucket of peanut butter? Will my five-gallon container of goldfish crackers still taste just as good in two years? And ... why is everyone shopping at the megastore overweight?

Efficiency and Convenience at a Price

Mass production of the twentieth-century industrial era convinced us that mass production on a large scale was the best thing for our economy and well-being. Abundance of food and mega portion sizes became a desirable goal.

Convenience—and eliminating the need to do any food preparation whatsoever—(other than perhaps heating something in the microwave) became the norm. Over the past few decades, we have learned that what is good for mass production is not good for our health. Efficiency means eliminating the art of cooking. Convenience means adding chemicals, additives, preservatives, artificial colors, and artificial flavors, and combining these ingredients all together in a cardboard box. Would Grandma have served this stuff to her children?

Eating on the Run

As nutrition and healthy eating take a backseat to other activities, our free time gets taken up driving from place to place and eating on the go. No time for a meal? Eat in the car! Often families spend dinner together in the minivan as we sit in traffic driving from work to soccer practice to music lessons. No wonder the latest Honda Odyssey minivan has seventeen cup holders! Now all I need is a drop-down tray table so I can also serve a meal as I drive!

No time for breakfast? Grab a meal-replacement shake or breakfast bar on the way out the door. Better yet, eat it in the car on the way to school or work! In the name of maximum efficiency, we have replaced the joy of eating a delicious and well-prepared meal with inhaling a prepackaged "health food product."

Vicious Cycle of Chronic Fatigue

Who isn't familiar with this cycle? It goes something like this, with individual variations:

We wake up exhausted until that first cup of coffee provides the caffeine we need to give our bodies a jolt. We're too tired to eat breakfast in the morning, but then midmorning hits and our craving for sugar kicks in so badly that it is nearly impossible to avoid eating a doughnut, pastry, scone, or sugar-coated cereal … and maybe washing it down with another cup of coffee or soda.

There isn't enough time to sit down to a healthy, fresh lunch, so we grab a fast-food meal and wolf it down in time to get back to work—full, but tired again by mid afternoon. The sugar and caffeine cravings then hit once again. By dinnertime, we are so hungry that we require a quick snack beforehand. We grab a takeout dinner or heat up a frozen convenience-food item and add a ready-made dessert. Nighttime TV includes more commercials for yet more convenience foods, stimulating us to snack while watching TV far too late into the night … so that we get up once again the next day fatigued with no appetite except for a morning cup of coffee.

It's Not Food; it's a Food Product

In the name of wholesome goodness, the food industry has bamboozled us into believing that much of what is sold is actually food, when in reality it is a "food product" at best. Who would believe the day would come in 2004 when we would lament the bankruptcy of the company <u>Interstate</u>

Bakeries, that gave us Wonder bread, Ho Hos, and RingDings? A powerful icon of the American way has gone by the wayside. Horrors!

Generations of children might grow up without the experience of coming home from school and eating the same mass-produced, preserved sugar fix that their parents did! My mother was genuinely saddened to hear that her grandchildren might miss out on this experience, which had been such a huge part of my childhood. The power of food-product marketing cannot be underestimated! Who would have dreamed that one day we would look back fondly at the day when 'real moms' used to mix Kool-Aid powder with sugar rather than grab a juice box?

The Toxic Food Environment in Which We Live

Dr. Kelly Brownell, a Yale University professor of nutrition and eating disorders who was a consultant for the film *Super Size Me*, has said in her book, *Food Fight*: "Americans live in a 'toxic food and physical inactivity environment,' which means that many Americans live in an environment that 'almost guarantees' that they become ill and diseased, and that although not all Americans will get sick, more and more of them will."

Some interesting fast-food trivia that the movie *Super Size Me*, (a 2004 documentary film during which the filmmaker subsists entirely on food and items purchased exclusively from McDonald's during a 30 day period) gave us included the following:

1. Each day, one in four Americans visits a fast-food establishment.
2. McDonald's alone feeds more than 46 million people a day. That number is larger than the entire population of Spain.
3. French fries are the most commonly consumed vegetable in America.
4. Only seven items on the McDonald's menu contain no sugar.

TV commercials, billboards, magazine and newspaper ads, and the ever-present food product deal at the grocery and convenience store tempt us to purchase and bring into our homes the modern-day food products engineered by today's food conglomeration empire. When grocery shopping with kids, who can resist the "two-for-one" box of cookies with Winnie the Pooh or Dora the Explorer or Bob the Builder on the label?

We train our kids early that this is the American way. We teach them at the preschool age that fast food is a special treat associated with a special toy. We permit the direct marketing of fast foods, snack foods, candy, sugar-coated cereals, and soda directly to our kids. Our kids take the bus to school when once walking to school would have been the norm. Many school districts have begun to eliminate physical education classes in order to increase classroom time. Some school cafeterias now come complete with soda and snack machines, where a hot lunch is often 'heat and eat' and no cooking or meal preparation actually takes place. Thus, physical activity and good nutrition become de-emphasized in a typical schoolchild's day

Fat Chance

Is it a surprise to anyone that as a society we eat too much, exercise too little, and therefore weigh too much? This trend has been going on for some time, and continues.

We have heard the message from many experts:

> The 2005 report *Preventing Childhood Obesity: Health in the Balance*, written by the Institute of Medicine and commissioned by Congress, calls for making the prevention of childhood obesity a national public health priority. According to the report, the rate of obesity over the past thirty years has more than doubled for preschool children ages two to five and adolescents ages twelve to nineteen; it has more than tripled for children aged six to eleven. Childhood obesity carries with it a number of serious health impli-

cations, including an increased risk for developing diabetes and other chronic conditions.

The Centers for Disease Control and Prevention offers the following statistics for the United States, 1999–2002:

- Percent of adults ages twenty and over who are overweight or obese: 65%
- Percent of adults ages twenty and over who are obese: 33% (compared with 23% in 1994)
- Percent of adolescents ages twelve to nineteen who are overweight: 15% (triple what the proportion was in 1980)
- Percent of children ages six to eleven who are overweight: 15% (triple what the proportion was in 1980)

Source: Health-E Stats http://www.cdc.gov/nchs/products/pubs/pubd/hestats/hestats.htm

Other published data from several sources including Centers for Disease Control and Prevention, *Journal of the American Medical Association, Pediatrics,* U.S. Department of Agriculture, *Lancet, Archives of Pediatrics and Adolescent Medicine,* Tufts University/Friedman School of Nutrition Science and Policy, Kaiser Family Foundation tell us this:

- Increase in childhood diabetes in the last twenty years from 1985–2005: tenfold increase
- Percent increase in soft drink intake per capita since the 1950s: 500%
- Percent of children who eat fast food on a given day: 30%
- Percent increase in children's obesity risk from one additional soft drink per day: 60%

- Percent of every U.S. food dollar spent on food eaten outside the home: 49%

(Source: Harvard Public Health Review: Spring 2006, p. 13)

Health Consequences

The Center for Chronic Disease Prevention and Health Promotion gives a list of physical ailments associated with being overweight. They include:

- High blood pressure
- High blood cholesterol
- Diabetes
- Heart disease
- Congestive heart failure
- Stroke
- Gallstones
- Gout
- Osteoarthritis
- Sleep apnea
- Some types of cancer (such as endometrial, breast, prostate, and colon)
- Complications of pregnancy
- Poor female reproductive health (such as menstrual irregularities, infertility, irregular ovulation)
- Bladder control problems (such as stress incontinence)

- Psychological disorders (such as depression, eating disorders, distorted body image, and low self-esteem).
- Others

Source: Center for Disease Control *http://www.cdc.gov/nccdphp/dnpa/obesity/consequences.htm*

What Can You Do about It?

This book will start you on your journey of nutritional awareness and change. It involves reexamining your approach to food and exercise and the value you place on you and your family's health. As one of my best friends is fond of saying, and I believe even Bill Gates would agree, "If you have your health, you've got everything!"

Your journey will consist of these steps:

- Learning about mindful eating, incorporating a more relaxed approach to your life, and finding pleasure and reward in eating healthy foods.
- Gaining awareness of outside influences and their impact on how much you eat.
- Understanding what food ingredients, food handling practices, and other damaging food processing practices to avoid.
- Developing a healthy relationship with food and exercise to improve your health and energy level.

Chapter 2:

Mindful Eating: Eating as if Your Life Depended on It!

He that won't be counseled can't be helped.
—Benjamin Franklin

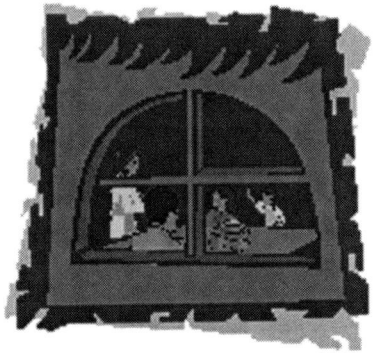

Objectives:
- What does it mean to eat mindfully?
- Why is mindful eating beneficial?
- How can I achieve mindful eating in my life? In my family's life?

Have you ever found yourself munching on something when you realized you really were not enjoying the food? I recall eating jelly beans that were attractively displayed on my coworker's desk. I just ate them because they were there. I did not actually realize I was eating them until after I had eaten several handfuls. Ironically, I do not even like jelly beans! Don't we all have a coworker or friend who keeps a constant supply of tempting, calorie-laden snack foods for the rest of us? Amusingly, these same people hardly touch the stuff; they just keep it out for the rest of us! This is a perfect example of eating mind*less*ly. Has this ever happened to you?

It is so easy to fall into the trap of eating food simply because it is there. Mindful eating includes being aware of eating; yet awareness is only one part of being mindful. The concept of mindful eating incorporates the atmosphere of the meal, the taste and smell of the food, the appreciation for the person who prepared the food, and your gratefulness for the garden in which the food was grown.

Mindless Eating: The Great American Pastime

In his book *Mindless Eating,* Brian Wansink, PhD, documents the years he has spent researching the eating of the average American. His research demonstrates that we are powerfully, though subconsciously, affected by environmental cues that control how much and what we eat. A few of the interesting conclusions from his research include:

- The smaller the plate, the less we will eat—this goes for dinner plates, as well as beverage containers. We will unwittingly eat more when served a larger portion, regardless of our hunger.

Strategy: Use a smaller dinner-plate size when serving at home. Serve small portions, and allow family members to go back for seconds.

- Dish out 20 percent less than you think you will want when you start to eat. Chances are, you won't even notice.
- The larger the volume of food is available, the more people eat. For example, people will eat more M&Ms out of a half-pound bag than if given the same volume of M&Ms in individual packets.

Strategy: Snacks should be portioned into one-hundred-calorie sizes, not taken from an open package.

- o Warehouse-club grocery shopping increases food consumption. We go there to buy large quantities at bargain prices. We may even buy substantially more than we need in order to stock up and have bountiful amounts of excess food at home. We know large containers cause us to dish out larger quantities of food, but what about the large containers of individually packaged food, such as the instant-oatmeal box with forty-eight packets?

According to Wansink's research, just having the items in our immediate environment—seeing them every time we open the cabinet door—gives us a cue to eat more of that product. And at the end, when we have eaten through a substantial portion, we are then motivated to continue eating more—just to finish it up.

Strategy: Sometimes, less is more. Buy food in reasonable volumes.

- o TV eating is a triple threat. For some, the TV is a cue to eat. It is a ritual—we turn on the TV, salivate, get a snack. When we watch TV, not only are we not paying attention to *what* we eat, we are unaware of *how much* we eat.

Strategy: Eat without distraction. If TV eating is a must-do ritual, dish out a small portion before you start TV watching. Limit eating to the kitchen or dining room.

In conclusion, reengineer your personal eating environment to optimize your eating habits without deprivation.

Enjoy eating as if it were a delightful journey. Being mindful incorporates many emotional and physical responses associated with having a meal. The goal of mindful eating is to help establish a positive relationship with food. When you are not mindful of the calories you eat (*mindless* eating), you tend to eat more throughout the day and weight gain becomes inevitable. Having an awareness of true hunger versus "just wanting some food" is crucial. Equally important is finding pleasure in food's flavor and appearance. Mindful eating is a rewarding goal.

Buddhist monk and author Thich Nhat Hanh speaks about mindful eating as a very pleasant event in the book, *For a Future to Be Possible: Commentaries on the Five Wonderful Precepts* (1993). He discusses how important it is to focus on putting the food in our mouth. He states that when eating a carrot, "don't put anything else into your mouth, like projects, your worries, and your fear, just put the carrot in."

Although eating on the run and multitasking in the name of efficiency are emphasized in today's world, healthy eating habits that require our attention and focus contribute to long-term success with winning eating habits. Engaging in a conscious eating pattern will be worth the effort. It is likely that food will take on a positive role in your life.

Challenges to Mindful Eating

Think back to the last time you ate a meal from an all-you-can-eat buffet. Did you experience indigestion? Do you remember feeling relaxed at the buffet? Were you concerned about getting your money's worth? Were you able to stop eating at the point when you were comfortably full, or did you find yourself overeating when faced with limitless quantities of a variety of foods?

Think back to the last time you ate in the car while driving. Eating in the car has become a mainstream mealtime activity, but not without consequences. How can we be mindful and relaxed and maximize digestion if we're wolfing down a meal in a traffic jam?

When we are stressed, our bodies respond with the following changes:

- Increased metabolism
- Rapid heart rate
- Elevated blood pressure
- Faster breathing rate
- Muscle tension

Eating while stressed is not ideal for digestion. If we are to digest our food properly and derive full nutritional value from the foods we eat, we need to approach meal times with serenity and find pleasure in what we are eating.

Rediscovering the Pleasure: Exercises in Mindful Eating

Try to simply eat. That is, shut off the television, close the magazine or newspaper, get out of the car, and just eat. Make the room enjoyable. Light a candle, dim the lights, and maybe turn on some relaxing music. Try to unwind. Be aware and conscious of the meal you intend to eat. Let eating be pleasurable, not a means to an end.

Plan a menu that appeals to you. Don't eat leftovers if you hate leftovers. Take a moment to think about what you and your children feel like eating. Menu planning makes meal preparation easier because you will have the food items necessary to make the meals you all enjoy, in the home and ready to use. You don't have to be a short-order cook, but do consider the preferences of those you are feeding.

Take note of food that has lovingly been made in your honor. Notice the color, the texture, and the balance. Feel good about putting food into your body. Do you feel good if you have a healthy, balanced, tasty meal in front of you? Yes, there is only one way to feel: gratefully satisfied.

Balance is essential when it comes to planning and eating a meal. Remember to be mindful when selecting when and what you are going to eat. Factor in your food preferences, your time constraints, and your personal energy level to take on the task. This will foster positive feelings associated with the meal and the final outcome of actually eating the meal.

Eating thoughtfully and consciously feels great when you practice it regularly. Keep in mind that your personal strategy for mindful eating may need to ebb and flow with the way each day unfolds. Paying more attention to where, what, and why you are eating can be a rewarding experience for you, your family, and your friends.

Achieving Relaxation

An important precursor to mindful eating requires achieving a calm state. There are many breathing techniques that can help, as described by Herbert Benson, a Harvard cardiologist well known for his mind-body studies. Some of these techniques are outlined in Benson's *The Wellness Book,* coauthored with Eileen M. Stuart, R.N. Benson found that repeating a word or phrase continuously in a melodic manner replaces the distressing thoughts that keep us tense during waking hours. Using the techniques outlined in his book results in a slower heart rate, lower blood pressure, and slower breathing.

Other ways to help take it down a notch include:

- avoid over scheduling yourself or your children
- learn how to say "no" to certain volunteer opportunities
- work off a list to help you stay focused on the important chores for the day
- incorporate outdoor activity (be one with nature)
- shut off the television and listen to more music.

Kids and Mindful Eating

As parents, it is our job to promote mindful eating strategies at home. Take time to stop for breakfast. Enjoy some nourishing foods together before going out into the real world. It is a great way to start to your day. How many children truly eat a nourishing breakfast before school? In my experience counseling children and their families, I have found that breakfast is often missed or replaced with a granola bar. Try to wake everyone up twenty minutes earlier than usual to allow for a less stressful transition into the day. This extra time will allow your family to enjoy a healthy breakfast together.

Meals eaten away from home also provide a challenge to promoting mindful eating. The typical school age child is most likely to find eating lunch in the school cafeteria a far cry from the optimal mindful eating experience. Lunchtime restrictions, as well as the typical cafeteria environment, make eating slowly in a relaxed manner close to impossible. At the middle school in my hometown, the kids are allowed twenty-one minutes for lunch. This twenty-one-minute lunch break includes buying the meal, finding a seat, and eating. By the time they sit down, my son estimates that the students have about five minutes before the 'Snack Shack'—a moving kiosk of snack foods—arrives. This initiates a ritual of kids dashing to get to the 'Snack Shack' line, again, and wasting more of their precious eating time to purchase a candy bar, chips, or a soda. When children bring their lunches, they do not waste unnecessary time in the lunch line. Try to encourage your child to bring lunch more often to allow some extra down time.

Tips for Promoting Mindful Eating with Your Kids

- Although hard to execute in today's busy world, do not hurry meals, but do not let kids dawdle either. Twenty minutes for mealtime is reasonable for a five-year-old or younger—longer for older kids.
- Sit with your kids, and eat the same foods they do.

- Bribing or rewarding with food could send the wrong message about food.
- If possible, serve meals "family style" so that each person can choose his or her own portion size. For small children, one tablespoon per age for each food is a good guide for portion size. (For those who need portion control, this method is not suggested. Rather, appropriate portions should be served, and seconds offered only if requested.)
- Let your kids help with menu planning and cooking.
- Encourage good table manners.
- Ask about the meal being served. Can the kids taste specific flavors?
- Discuss where the food came from. This will bring forth a different thought process about the food and possibly a greater appreciation for the food as well.
- Encourage everyone to chew slowly and thoughtfully.
- Pack a brown bag lunch as often as possible to allow for more eating time for you and your kids.
- Consider picking apples, strawberries, or blueberries when in season. This is a great family activity that teaches children about the fruit, where it comes from, and how much better it tastes when fresh.

Take Action: Practice Mindful Eating and Relaxation

- Plan to eat a quiet, nourishing breakfast with your family one day this week.
- Light candles at the dinner table. Add a bouquet of flowers. Put on relaxing background music.
- Shut off the television during *all* meals.

- Have everyone discuss dinner menus for the week ahead, and plan meals together that appeal to all family members.
- Sign a petition with local families to discuss the school lunch program in your hometown. Discuss how much time your children have to eat their lunches. Is it enough time to allow for mindful eating? Does the school serve unhealthy food choices in vending machines? What other options can your school system consider?
- Try breathing techniques that promote relaxation. Consider meditation or yoga to bring peace to your soul.
- Have each person at the dinner table discuss the best thing that happened to him or her that day.
- Don't forego your favorite decadent dessert, but choose a smaller portion than you usually do. Chew slowly, without engaging in any other activities.

Sometimes we are just plain bored and truly not hungry. If boredom makes you reach for the snacks in your home, consider trying the following activities to distract your mind from food cravings:

- Be at one with nature. Enjoy a walk outside.
- Listen to your favorite music.
- Dance.
- Take a bubble bath. Include low lighting and fragrant candles.
- Play on the computer.
- Call a friend.
- Sing.
- Listen to a sound machine (with a bubbling brook or ocean waves).
- Have your children fill an "idea jar" with activities they could do when they're bored (for example, make a collage, play with clay, read a book, or build with *Legos*).

Chapter 3:
Kids Keeping Pace in a Fast-Food World

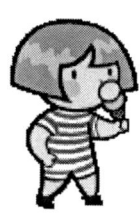 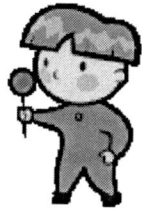

Twenty years from now you will be more disappointed by the things you didn't do than by the ones you did do. So throw off the bowlines. Sail away from the safe harbor. Catch the trade winds in your sails. Explore. Dream. Discover.
—Mark Twain

> Objectives:
> - How can I increase nutrition awareness in my child?
> - How can I model healthy habits for my children?
> - How can I counteract the harmful effects of fast-food marketing?

As a dietitian, one of the most commonly asked questions parents have is this, "How can I get my kids to eat a healthy diet? How can I get my kids to eat more fruits, vegetables, low-fat dairy products, or whole grains, and less unhealthy snack foods?"

Moms and dads use many methods to combat this eternal struggle, many of which create a battle of wills between parents and kids. I classify a number of approaches as follows:

The Food Chemistry Method. Mom or Dad becomes a professional food chemist and experiments with different ways of secretly hiding vegetables in various preparations—black bean brownies, cauliflower mashed potatoes, and the like. I find this method to be particularly popular among very creative parents, who will swap recipes that employ various food-hiding strategies.

The Fear of Starvation and Debilitating Weakness Strategy. Mom or Dad fears that the kid(s) will not receive an adequate amount of nutrients, which may compromise any number of activities, from schoolwork to athletic endeavors. Thus, children are expected to finish each and every serving of the appropriate food categories painstakingly prepared and carefully served at each meal.

Of course, our kids are not likely to buy into this expectation one bit and will likely come up with all kinds of diversions to get around this effort. Some diversions my kids have tried on me are "Daddy said I don't have to eat it" or "I only need to eat my number" (meaning they only need to eat the number of bites equal to their age) or "But Grandma lets us have Pepsi and candy for dinner at her house."

Some moms or dads will follow their kids around and actually try to get food into their mouths. Other moms will simply say "I give up" and hand the kid a carton of chocolate milk or some such other "meal replacement" beverage.

"Do as I Say, Not as I do" Strategy. My kids know that once it is bedtime, teeth have been brushed, and the lights are out, there is to be no further snacking. The kitchen is closed to everyone—except for Daddy. My husband loves nothing more than to snack at night in front of the TV. This can only be done after the kids are in bed; if they had any idea this was going on, they would be right there with him, watching TV and eating snacks late into the night. This, and other bad eating behaviors we hope our kids never pick up, will be hard to hide forever. Once they are known, they are sure to be emulated.

The Nutrition Deficit Disorder: Be aware of the importance of managing your kids' environment.

The impact of mass marketing geared toward our children cannot be underestimated. According to Susan Linn's book *Consuming Kids*, mass marketing to children is a $15 billion industry. Much of those billions go toward marketing *unhealthy*, processed food directly to children through TV commercial advertising. Here are some of the hair-raising statistics she provides:

- It is estimated that kids who watch Saturday morning television see an average of one food commercial every five minutes—all of which advertise unhealthy foods.
- Food tie-ins to TV characters—*Rugrats* pictured on Kraft Macaroni & Cheese boxes, *SpongeBob SquarePants* shown on cracker boxes, *Winnie the Pooh* featured on graham crackers, *Sesame Street* characters pictured on juice boxes—lure children and their parents into choosing and eating food associated with their favorite shows or movies.
- According to Linn, "Food advertising works. Children's request for food products, misperceptions about nutrition and increased caloric intake have been shown to be linked to television advertising."
- The incidence if obesity is highest among children who watch four or more hours of television a day.
- Among teenagers, the incidence of obesity increases by 2 percent for every additional hour of television watched.

Our Strategies

Limit your kids' exposure to unhealthy food commercials. The American Academy of Pediatrics (www.aap.org) gives these guidelines for 'screen time' which applies to computers, video games, movies, and TV;

- No TV for children ages two or younger.
- For older children, no more than one to two hours per day of educational, nonviolent programs. The combined time for all media activities shouldn't exceed 2 hours.

Although this may be unrealistic for many families, you can use TV viewing as a way to develop critical thinking skills in your kids. For example, get up with your kids some Saturday morning and take a closer look at the cartoons they're watching. Use the following worksheet to analyze the use of marketing to promote junk foods, and talk about it with your kids.

TV Viewing Worksheet

Date:_____

Time started:_____

Time stopped:_____

Network:_____

Foods eaten during TV watching time:_____
_____

WHO
Who is marketing the product to you? What manufacturer/company?

Who is the target audience?

WHAT
Count the number of commercials for food.

Count the types of food commercials for:

- ☐ Grains (breads, cereals, pasta, rice)
- ☐ Fruits or Juices
- ☐ Vegetables
- ☐ Protein sources
- ☐ Dairy Products
- ☐ Others:

How often are healthy, nutritious foods advertised? How often are unhealthy foods advertised?

WHEN
When do the commercials suggest that you eat these foods?

WHERE
Where do the commercials suggest you eat these foods?

HOW
How do the commercials make you feel about eating those foods? Does it make you feel hungry to watch these ads? Do you think that you will want to buy those foods based on the ads you saw?

Be conscious of the power advertising has on you when you are choosing food for your kids. Just because your son really likes dinosaurs right now, does he really need to have dinosaur-shaped chicken nuggets for dinner? Do you really want to continue buying them on a regular basis until the dinosaur phase of his life is over? What about his sister who doesn't like dinosaurs but does like Dora the Explorer? Are you going to spend your time looking for an alternate shape of chicken nugget for her dinner? An innocent desire to please a child can backfire as one gets sucked into the mass marketing whirlwind.

When you do purchase foods with packaging aimed at kids, take the food out of the package when you get home and put it in a clear, plastic container. You are not depriving your children of their favorite snacks, but they will likely eat less of it without the enticing packaging. This works so well in my family that it's become a habit for me to routinely take all snack foods out of the packaging and store them in clear storage containers. Somehow, without the flashy packaging, my family eats less snack items—especially in one sitting.

Teach your kids about mass marketing. Use a trip to the grocery store to increase your children's brand awareness, and use their desire to purchase certain foods as an opportunity to teach them about advertising. Explain the concept of junk food. Point out that the reason their favorite character is on the box is because the people who make that product want families to buy it—not because the food is necessarily good for them.

When my son was three and we went grocery shopping together, we used to have this conversation often. He would say, "They just want us to buy *all* of [whatever product was of interest at that moment] until we have no more money." And in reply I would say, "Can you believe it?"

Interpret nutrition in the news as a family. Ask yourself the following questions the next time you hear or read a news story on a nutrition topic:

- Beware of phrases like "startling revelation," "now we know," or "this study proves" used to describe findings. They are often used to create sensationalism.
- Does the article or news story imply that all other previous nutrition findings are obsolete or no longer valid on this topic?
- Does the article or news story cite credible references or the scientific journal in which the research was published? Is an opposing point of view included?
- Does the nutrition topic apply to you or your family?
- Does the news story or article warrant a change in eating habits? Or, before changing your lifestyle, is it worth noting until additional research supports or reinforces the conclusion?
- How can you learn more about this topic from a credible source?

Eat by example. Your kids will model your behavior. If, like my husband, you enjoy snacking while watching TV late at night, eventually your kids will catch on! If eating in front of the TV is a must, consider dishing out a portion size to eat, rather than bringing the entire snack package with you to the screen.

Serve the family meal on a platter. One way of serving your family, rather than putting portions directly on the plate or even in multiple serving bowls, is to display the entire meal attractively on a large platter. Each person serves him or herself from the large platter in a gesture evoking times of old. This will not work for the very young, but it will provide older kids the opportunity to make healthy food choices and determine their own portion sizes. Although you have chosen the menu, they will enjoy serving themselves. Somehow a meal becomes more intimate this way, with everyone partaking of the same source.

For families who find portion control at meals a challenge, it is best to dish out an appropriate serving size on each plate, and permit second helpings only if requested.

Build your own meal. You can serve build-your-own meals to give your kids healthy choices while recognizing their individual preferences. Possibilities include the following:

Baked potato with toppings. Toppings might include broccoli (precooked), grated cheese, chili, sour cream, chopped olives, chives, chopped tomatoes, low-fat sour cream, and bacon bits made from low-fat turkey bacon.

Pizza. Topping suggestions include fresh, chopped pineapple; homemade bacon bits from low-fat turkey bacon; low-fat turkey pepperoni; olives; fresh herbs such as oregano, basil, or chives; fresh tomato slices or sun dried tomatoes; and goat cheese or other varieties of cheese.

Chef salad. You might offer fresh greens, low-fat deli meats, low-fat cheese slices, carrots, radishes, mushroom slices, sliced summer squash, pea pods chopped boiled egg, pickle slices, sunflower seeds, croutons, sprouts, olives, sweet corn cut from the cob, and pepper slices.

Use portion control. It is never too soon for kids to learn about appropriate serving sizes. As soon as your kids are old enough to count, a good question to ask is "How many would you like?" (as in how many raisins, pretzels, crackers, nuts, scoops of granola, and so on, they plan to eat in that sitting). This is a great way to reinforce counting for beginners and to get your kids to think about what amount they will be eating before they eat it. You have taught them the habit of preplanning their snack—and reinforced counting—all at once!

When in doubt, read the label for the portion size. Although sizes may often seem remarkably small, they are real portions intended as guidelines for consumption. See if you eat less ice cream if you actually dish out a half cup rather than eating it straight out of the carton. I bet you will. Try it! Just remember, an entire sleeve of *Oreos* or *Ritz* crackers is not a serving size! Can you believe it?!

Make meals together with your family. I have to admit that on some days, it took a lot of patience to include my one-, three-, and four-year-olds in the kitchen when making dinner. I had to keep reminding myself that in addition to being in my way, they were indirectly receiving a host of valuable educational benefits. These included:

- **An appreciation for food preparation.** Perhaps one day they may even have enough skill to make a meal for themselves!
- **Exposure to reading instructions and following them.** Even those who are too young to read can follow along as you read a recipe. They can also understand that words not only can be used to tell a story, but can convey other important information as well.
- **Early math and use of fractions.** Using measuring cups and spoons, determining the number of ounces needed from a can, doubling recipes, identifying degrees on the oven temperature—all offer exposure to using math in a practical way.
- **Basic science.** The use of leavening agents, yeast, liquids that blend and separate, water's properties as a gas, liquid, or a solid—you can discuss all of these matters with your child as you are cooking together.
- **Simple conservation.** It isn't often that we have a chance to have a conversation with our children. Preparing a meal together can offer that opportunity.
- **Teamwork.** This may be one of your child's first opportunities to work on a group project, with the end result being dinner. Being able to work as a member of a team is a skill that will serve your child well in any situation.
- **Passing on culture, heritage, and traditions**. Dinner preparation is a chance to pass on your culinary heritage to your children. Get Grandma's recipe for her secret casserole, and pass it on!
- **Menu planning**. Letting your family members participate in menu planning can help picky eaters feel empowered and gives your family some responsibility for what is on the table that night. I find that

giving everybody a dinner choice each week (within reason) cuts down on the number of uneaten meals and negative commentary.
- o **Etiquette.** This is a chance to teach your kids how to set a dinner table, how to use a napkin, and other table manners. They will be ready for the Ritz in no time!

Take Action

- Try viewing TV together and discussing the content of food advertising.
- The next time you are grocery shopping with your kids, point out marketing techniques as a way to jump-start a discussion.
- Try making a meal together. Everyone should participate in cleanup!
- Make an old family recipe that has been passed down from a previous generation.
- Find the portion sizes on the labels of the items you eat this week. Serve yourself and your kids accordingly.
- Take the following survey to assess you and your family's healthy habits.

Healthy Habits Quiz:

Do you and your family …	Yes	No	Sometimes
Have regularly scheduled mealtimes at home?	○	○	○
Eat meals together at least once a day?	○	○	○
Plan snacks?	○	○	○
Tailor portion sizes to each person's needs?	○	○	○
Eat three meals every day?	○	○	○

Do you and your family …	Yes	No	Sometimes
Try to make mealtimes enjoyable?	○	○	○
Avoid making everyone eat everything on their plate?	○	○	○
Make meals last more than fifteen minutes?	○	○	○
Eat only in designated areas of the house?	○	○	○
Avoid using food to punish or reward?	○	○	○
Enjoy physical activities together once or twice a week?	○	○	○

"Yes" = 2 points
"Sometimes" = 1 point
"No" = 0 points

Your total score is: ☐

If your total score is:

20–22—Your family is on the right track. Use this guide for additional healthy eating and physical activity ideas.

13–19—Your family is doing well, but could work on areas where you answered "no"/"sometimes."

12 or lower—This guide should be very helpful as you try to help your child reach a healthy weight.

© 2003, American Dietetic Association. *If Your Child Is Overweight: A Guide for Parents,* 2nd Ed.

Chapter 4:

Balancing the Plate: Serving Up Variety and Proportion

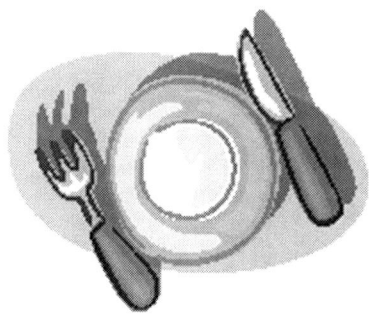

You will never plough a field if you only turn it over in your mind.
—Irish Proverb

> Objectives:
> - What proportions make up the optimal meal?
> - What does a "balanced" plate include?
> - Why is water important?

Balance is the key ingredient to a successful nutrition plan. Eating too much of one nutrient and not enough of the many others that are essential for good health does the body little good. Variety truly is the spice of life! Menu planning is vital to managing a healthy diet. Choosing carbohydrates that contain fiber (e.g., whole-grain breads vs. white bread), and adequate protein is a good start. Portion control is also important. I often tell the clients that I counsel on good nutrition, "It is not what you are eating, it is how much." Yes, you can eat too many apples! A whole bag of pretzels, although fat free, is too much. Always balance your plate.

The following diagram provides a simple guideline for the optimal combination of food on your plate.

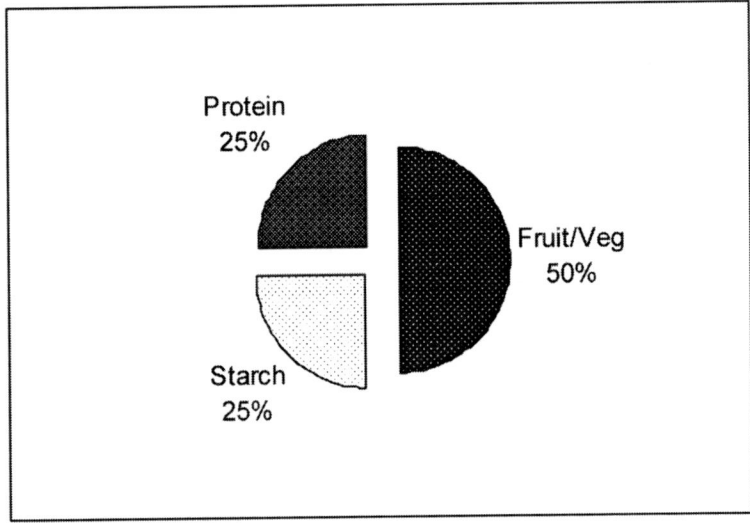

- Protein will be detailed later in this chapter; however, here is a sample of great protein choices: chicken, fish, turkey, lean beef, tofu, eggs, cheese, and beans (such as kidney, black, pinto, etc.). An easy tip for protein foods is to keep the portion to the size of the palm of your hand.
- Although given a bad rap, fats are a required element of a healthy diet, particularly fats or oils derived from plants or fish.
- Fruits and vegetables supply your body with a variety of vitamins, minerals, and disease-fighting nutrients called antioxidants. The key to this group is to choose a variety, ideally a rainbow of colors.
- Carbohydrates, often referred to as "starches", will also be detailed later in this chapter, but here is a quick list of great choices: brown rice, potatoes, peas, corn, pasta, and whole-grain breads and cere-

als. An easy guide for these foods is to keep the portion size to about the size of your fist.
- Meeting your body's fluid needs is also an important component of achieving nutritional balance. Although largely ignored by most nutrition guidelines, we emphasize it here.

Following this simple diagram above is an easy yet effective way to manage your distribution of protein, carbohydrate, and fruit/vegetable intake. Let's take a closer look at these important components.

Protein

What we are normally served in a restaurant or even at home bears no resemblance to the portion sizes listed on the side of a label or what food references use as a "serving" size—particularly when it comes to meat. For any kind of meat, whether beef, chicken, pork, or fish, three ounces is considered *one* serving. Astonishingly, three ounces of meat is approximately the size of a deck of cards! This means that a serving size of meat would fit into the shape below—21/2" x 31/2" or the size of a deck of cards:

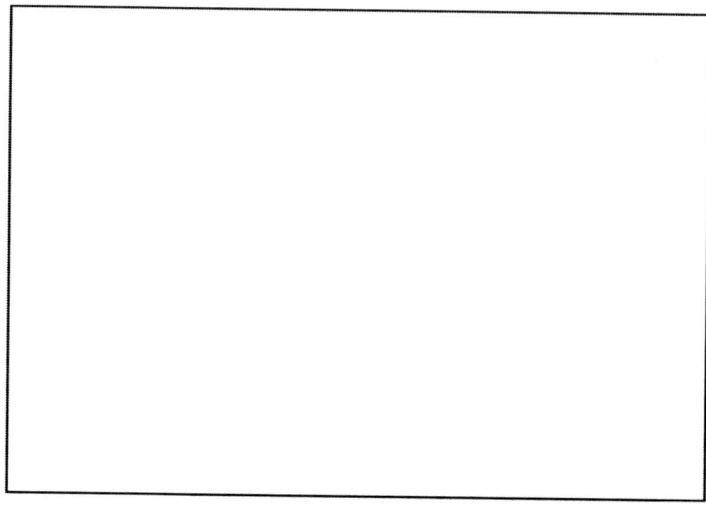

We can leave most of the meat served on the plate of a typical restaurant and still be meeting our protein needs! In fact, the American Heart Association recommends no more than six ounces of *lean* meat per day for all healthy Americans.

Protein needs vary by gender, weight, height, and age. By reducing meat portions to the recommended size, additional protein needs to come from nonmeat sources such as beans, low-fat dairy products, nuts, soy products like tofu, or eggs.

When caloric intake is adequate, protein helps maintain muscle. As muscle tissue helps burn calories, maintaining adequate amounts of protein in our diet is essential. Without adequate protein, our body will use muscle, in addition to fat, as fuel. Fortunately, obtaining adequate protein is not a concern in our country as it is in many third-world countries. When starvation is self-imposed, as often happens when dieters adhere to a strict calorie limit, and far too little calories and protein are consumed, muscle breakdown does occur. The breakdown of muscle makes a dieter's body less efficient at burning calories in the long term, as muscle tissue is far more efficient at burning calories than fat tissue. (*See chapter 11 for more information on exercise and metabolism.*)

Fat

Although fat gets a bad reputation, it does play an essential role in our bodies. It performs some of the following functions:

- Maintains healthy skin and hair.
- Cushions vital organs.
- Protects the body from temperature extremes.
- Carries fat-soluble nutrients and fat-soluble vitamins: A, D, E.
- Acts as a component in hormone formation.

Fats are made up of basic units called fatty acids. Each type of fat has a mixture of fatty acids and can be categorized as one of the following: saturated fat, *trans* saturated fat, monounsaturated fat, or polyunsaturated fat.

The American Heart Association (www. americanheart.org) describes the four types of fats this way:

Saturated fat tends to be solid at room temperature and is found primarily in animal products such as cream, whole milk, butter, cheese, ice cream, and fatty meats such as beef, sausage, and poultry skin. Additionally, it is found in cocoa butter, a prime ingredient in chocolate. Saturated fat increases LDL (bad) cholesterol and total cholesterol, increasing the risk of heart disease and stroke.

Monounsaturated fat tends to be liquid at room temperature. Food sources include olives, olive oil, avocado, nuts and nut butters, and canola oil. Research suggests that a diet rich in these fats may lower LDL (bad) cholesterol and thereby decrease heart disease risk. These fats also maintain good cholesterol (HDL) levels.

Polyunsaturated fat tends to be liquid at room temperature and is the primary source of essential fatty acids that our body is unable to produce on its own. Sources include corn, safflower, sunflower, and soybean oils. Research suggests that this fat will lower LDL cholesterol; however, it may also lower HDL cholesterol (the good cholesterol).

Omega-3 fatty acids are one of the polyunsaturated fats. They are found in the greatest quantities in fatty fish such as salmon, halibut, tuna, mackerel, trout, sardines, eel, and herring. Because omega-3s have such a beneficial effect on cardiovascular health, the American Heart Association recommends eating fish one to two times per week. Some plants, such as flaxseed, arugula, and walnuts, also contain omega-3s. Ongoing research will determine whether plant-based omega-3s have the same beneficial effect as omega-3s found in fish. Incidentally, new research shows that free-range animal products such as beef, chicken, and eggs tend to have a higher proportion of omega-3s, much like the farm animals consumed by earlier farming generations. (**The Omega Principle** Some Fish Fats Protect the Heart. What If They Could Also Treat Your Brain? Washington Post 2003)

***Trans* fatty acids** are produced as a by-product of the *hydrogenation* process, in which liquid oils are converted to a hardened solid, thereby increasing stability and shelf life. *Trans* fatty acids can also be produced when foods are deep-fried. *Trans* fats raise LDL (bad) cholesterol and may also lower HDL (good) cholesterol, raising the risk for a heart attack or stroke. The American Heart Association recommends limiting intake to no more than 1 percent of total calories, which translates to about one to two grams for most Americans. There are no health benefits to *trans* fats in the diet.

Fat truly is essential in the diet. Attention all of you gals with a fat-free salad dressing packet in your purse: one recent study found that regular, or full-fat, salad dressings helped the body absorb the nutrients in the salad far better than light or fat-free varieties (*American Journal of Clinical Nutrition*, Vol. 80 (2), 396–403, August 2004).

Fruits/Vegetables

Colorful fruits and vegetables contain the bulk of the important vitamins, minerals, and antioxidants (healthy disease-fighters) our body needs. A *daily* diet rich in fruits and vegetables is vital for good health. Unfortunately, that fruit roll-up is not a fruit, and an occasional banana will not meet your nutritional needs!

Carbohydrates

Carbohydrates provide our body with energy. They additionally help the body make serotonin, a brain chemical that is important in mood regulation. Carbohydrates can be refined or unrefined. When a carbohydrate is refined, it has been processed, meaning the bran, the fiber, and most of the vitamins and minerals and have been removed. Processing results in a bland, white product with a long shelf life, and a long shelf life is a desirable end product for food manufacturers. This is one of the reasons mass produced bread stays "fresh" longer than a few days. The consumer, however, is the one who loses—that is, we lose out on the nutrients that nature intended.

Our body uses all types of carbohydrates similarly, although we digest carbohydrates that contain fiber at a slower rate. Some people seem to be more efficient at utilizing carbohydrates than others. Some studies such as the article "Association between Carbohydrate Intake and Serum Lipids" published in the Journal of the American College of Nutrition, Vol. 25, No. 2, 155–163 (2006) suggests that diets high in refined carbohydrates increase plasma triglycerides, which are a form of fat in our bloodstream that, when elevated, increase the risk of heart disease.

Another concern with diets high in refined carbohydrates is their effect on the important hormone insulin. Insulin prevents the level of sugar in our blood from getting too high. When our bodies no longer respond to insulin effectively, we develop what is called "insulin resistance'" or "glucose intolerance"—the first step toward developing type 2 diabetes.

In addition to whole-wheat bread and whole-grain cereals, a whole world of whole grains is waiting for you to try at your local grocer or natural food store. Give some a try!

Your carbohydrate portion should be about one-fourth of your plate, approximately the size of your fist. Keep in mind that your child should consume a fist sized portion, Dad should consume a portion the size of his fist, and so on.

Fiber

Fiber is classified into two types: soluble fiber and insoluble fiber. Insoluble fiber is found primarily in foods that contain whole wheat and bran. This type of fiber is essential in lowering the risk of diverticulosis, a common intestinal disorder found in people living in industrialized countries like our own. Soluble fiber, on the other hand, is helpful in lowering cholesterol levels, which in turn lowers the risk of heart disease. Additionally, soluble fiber helps our bodies regulate blood sugar levels. Soluble fiber is found in oatmeal, oat bran, legumes, and fruit. Both soluble and insoluble fibers contribute to satiety, or the sense of feeling full, and consequently can be helpful in controlling weight. Both kinds of fiber maintain regularity, preventing constipation.

Because fiber is something few of us get enough of (most Americans top off at fifteen grams/day,) recommended targets and ways to increase fiber are listed here. Aim for the following targets:

Total Fiber, Ages 1 Through 18 Years in grams per day (g/d)

Children	
1–3 years	19 g/d of Total Fiber
4–8 years	25 g/d of Total Fiber
Boys	
9–13 years	31 g/d of Total Fiber
14–18 years	38 g/d of Total Fiber
Girls	
9–13 years	26 g/d of Total Fiber
14–18 years	26 g/d of Total Fiber

Total Fiber, Ages 19 Years and Older

Men	
19–30 years	38 g/d of Total Fiber
31–50 years	38 g/d of Total Fiber
51–70 years	30 g/d of Total Fiber
> 70 years	30 g/d of Total Fiber
Women	
19–30 years	25 g/d of Total Fiber
31–50 years	25 g/d of Total Fiber
51–70 years	21 g/d of Total Fiber
> 70 years	21 g/d of Total Fiber

Source: Dietary Reference Intakes for Energy, Carbohydrate, Fiber, Fat, Fatty Acids, Cholesterol, Protein, and Amino Acids (Macronutrients), 2005 Food and Nutrition Board (FNB) of the National Academy of Sciences

How much fiber am I getting?

Here's a quick way to estimate your daily fiber intake:

Estimating Daily Fiber Intake	Servings	Average Fiber Content, Grams
Multiply the number of servings from each category by the average amount of fiber, and total the amount.	Fruits and vegetables	1.5
	Refined grains (white bread, pasta)	1.0
	Whole grains	2.5
	Legumes, nuts, seeds, high-fiber cereals, one-half cup	8

Ways to Increase Fiber in Your Diet

Breakfast

- Make hot cereal such as old-fashioned (not instant) oatmeal, wheat flakes, and seven-grain cereal part of your kids' morning meals.
- Add granola (see recipe), wheat germ, flaxseed meal, bran flakes, and fresh fruit on top of hot/cold cereal or yogurt.
- Choose cold cereals made with whole grains.
- Forego the *Bisquick* and make pancakes with whole-grain or buckwheat pancake mix and top with apples, berries, sliced bananas, or raisins.
- Alternatively, consider making banana or pumpkin pancakes. Simply add one mashed banana or one-third cup canned pumpkin to your favorite pancake mix.
- Serve whole-grain waffles topped with fruit.
- Buy whole-grain bagels, whole-wheat pita bread, or whole-grain English muffins.

Lunch and Dinner

- Make sandwiches with whole-grain bread, whole-wheat pita bread, or whole-wheat rollups.
- Try 100% whole-wheat hot dog buns and hamburger rolls.
- Use whole-grain spaghetti and other pastas, instead of white. Make this transition slowly by adding some whole-grain pasta to your white pasta and slowly increasing the proportion over time.
- Instead of white rice, serve wild or brown rice with meals. (In the frozen food sections of *Trader Joe's* and *Whole Foods*, you can find precooked brown rice. All you have to do is reheat it.)
- Spice up salads with berries, almonds, chickpeas, cooked artichokes, and beans (kidney, black, navy, or pinto).

- Use whole-grain (corn or whole-wheat) soft taco shells or tortillas to make burritos or wraps. Fill them with eggs and cheese for breakfast; turkey, cheese, lettuce, tomato, and light dressing for lunch; and beans, salsa, taco sauce, and cheese for dinner.
- Include fresh fruit as part of your child's lunch. Pears, apples, bananas, oranges, and berries are all high in fiber and pack easily in a school lunch.

Hydration: Is Your Glass Half Full?

We often have that daily urge for a coffee break yet neglect the one essential fluid that best meets our bodies' needs: water. The symptoms—fatigue, dry skin, dizziness, difficulty concentrating, and the telltale physiologic sign of dark yellow urine—are all indicators that our body needs a big glass of water.

Our bodies are 60 percent water; we cannot survive without it. Water helps the body eliminate waste, transport sugar to working muscles, and regulate heat. Without adequate hydration, you may experience chronic fatigue, lack of endurance, headaches, and a lack of mental clarity. Do you experience any of those symptoms midday? Often we grab a snack when actually our bodies are craving water.

How much fluid should you drink?

Although the first sign of dehydration is thirst, your body has already lost approximately two cups of fluid by the time that sensation is triggered. With as little as a 5 percent loss of body fluid, one can begin to experience headaches, fatigue, confusion, reduced quantity and darkening of urine, and an elevated heart rate. Although the often-quoted guideline of eight eight-ounce glasses per day is not a mandatory physiologic requirement, it is an excellent goal to strive for. In fact, the Institute of Medicine report on **Dietary Reference Intakes: Water, Potassium, Sodium, Chloride, and Sulfate, 2004** did not specify exact requirements for water, but set general recommendations for women at approximately 2.7 liters (91 ounces) of total water—from all beverages and foods—each day, and men an average of approximately 3.7 liters (125 ounces daily) of total water.

Increase fluids if you are sick with diarrhea and/or vomiting, which results in greater fluid loss. Fever or an increase in body temperature will lead to water loss and increase your need for more fluids. Exercising also increases fluid needs. A good guideline is to drink at least eight ounces of fluid, ideally water, prior to exercise and consume fluids during exercise if exercising for longer than an hour.

Although many fortified waters, sports drinks, and marketing for other beverages suggest that they are superior to water, water alone is the best fluid for rehydration. For workouts lasting less than two hours, water is the preferred choice.

For the endurance athlete, a sports drink may offer the following advantages:

- Added glucose (sugar) gives additional calories the body can use as fuel. However, most of us are trying to burn up calories through a workout, and adding them back with a sports drink is counterproductive.
- Added electrolytes (namely, sodium and potassium) are needed for the high-performance athlete working up a drenching sweat exceeding five to ten pounds per day (or 3% of body weight) for several consecutive days, or for athletes competing for longer than six to eight hours. However, the rest of us can replenish our sodium and potassium stores easily at our next meal.

In summary, good nutrition involves balance. Foods work together along with adequate hydration to make us feel energized and enhance our health. Try to find balance in your food choices. Be adventurous with the many foods available to you. Choose the fat and protein sources in your diet wisely. Eat well. Hydrate. Feel your best.

Take Action: On Balance

- Check your dinner plate. Is it balanced? Does it contain 50 percent fruits and vegetables, 25 percent starch, and 25 percent protein?
- How does it feel to eat a meal balanced in this way? Do you feel different after consciously choosing a meal prepared with this composition?
- Be conscious of having a protein and unrefined carbohydrate source together when having a meal or a snack.

Sample menu items to help incorporate protein-rich foods with high-fiber carbohydrates:

- Eat whole-grain cereal (two grams or more of fiber/serving) and low-fat milk.
- Serve whole-grain cereal with nonfat or low-fat yogurt.
- Toast a whole-wheat English muffin and top with two tablespoons of all-natural peanut butter.
- Enjoy whole-grain waffles topped with yogurt and sliced bananas.
- Make a sandwich out of whole-grain bread or a pita. Fill with baby greens, sliced turkey, and a splash of Italian dressing.
- Toss a salad with carrots, tomatoes, romaine lettuce, kidney beans or chickpeas, a sprinkle of reduced-fat cheese, and light dressing.
- Try sautéing sliced pears and walnuts with a small amount of olive oil. Once slightly browned, put on top of spring greens, and add a small amount of blue cheese and vinaigrette-style dressing.

Take Action: On Fats

- Use olive and canola oils as your primary fat sources.
- Incorporate polyunsaturated fats (soybean, corn, safflower, and sunflower oils) daily to provide essential fatty acids.
- Choose nuts as a fiber, protein, and healthy fat source. Add to cereals, salads, or snacks such as trail mix.
- Quick tip: purchase a *Misto* oil spray bottle. Fill three-quarters full with olive oil and one-quarter soybean, sunflower, or safflower oil to provide monounsaturated and essential fatty acids via polyunsaturated fats. Use for spraying salad greens, oiling a pan for cooking, etc.
- Avoid using solid fats; they tend to be high in saturated or *trans* fats.
- Cook with oils as opposed to solid fats when possible. (For example, there is no need to add butter or margarine to rice pilaf. Use a small amount of oil instead.)
- Choose butter blends instead of regular butter, or make your own by first softening a stick of unsalted organic butter. Put it in a blender or mixer with a whisk attachment. Beat until whipped, and then slowly add one-half cup canola or light olive oil while whipping the butter to aerate it. Now you have your own blended butter. You can even make your own flavored butters by adding herbs to make herb butter, honey to make honey butter, or cinnamon or maple syrup to make a sweet butter.
- Instead of baking a potato and filling it with real butter, try roasting potatoes that you have drizzled with olive oil and herb seasoning.
- Try grilling vegetables on an outdoor grill on medium heat or roasting vegetables in the oven at 450 degrees until they have reached the desired level of roasting. Drizzle with olive oil and seasonings such as Italian herbs or sea salt, pepper, and minced garlic. Yum!

- Try to consume omega-3-rich fish one to two times a week. These fish include salmon, tuna, mackerel, or bluefish.
- Add plant sources of omega-3 fatty acids such as arugula, walnuts, and flaxseed (use milled or meal, not full seed, as it is better absorbed by the body).
- Avoid deep-fried foods or foods with *trans fatty* acids.
- Substitute low-sodium, low-fat chicken broth in place of butter in recipes such as mashed potatoes and pasta dishes (see recipe).
- Use ground flaxseeds in muffin and bread recipes, or simply use it as a topping on yogurt or your favorite cereal.(See recipes for how-to's.)
- Use salad dressing made primarily of oil and vinegar blends. Avoid creamy ranch and blue cheese; they often contain unhealthy fats.

Take Action: On Hydration

- Bring a reusable water bottle with you for your ride to and from work.
- Keep a cup of water at your work site or desk.
- Purchase reusable water bottles and keep in your refrigerator for a quick grab and go.
- Try canned seltzer waters. Keep on hand for variety.
- Bring decaffeinated tea to work, and have it for your afternoon break.
- Serve water for yourself and family at every meal.
- Consume water-laden fruits and vegetables such as watermelon, cucumbers, and celery.

Chapter 5:

Healthy Eating for All: A Look at the 2005 USDA Food Pyramid Guidelines

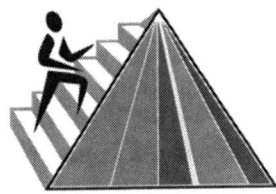

You will never find time for anything. If you want time, you make it.
—Charles Buxton

Objectives:
- How does the USDA food pyramid guidelines play a role in good nutrition for me and my family?

The U.S. Department of Agriculture's (USDA) new food pyramid, presented in 2005, gave us more specific guidelines for healthy eating. Despite the controversy that it inspired—that the USDA was adversely affected by powerful lobbyists from the fast-food and sugar industries, among others—it was a step in the right direction. Applying these guidelines to our own eating habits will help most of us consuming a standard American diet to be healthier. You can find more information at the USDA Web site: www.mypyramid.gov.

Why Should We Care?

Besides truly being the product of our genes and environment, and to repeat the adage "you are what you eat," an important question needs to be answered: why should we care about what scientific experts and policymakers recommend we eat?

According to the USDA, "the Dietary Guidelines for Americans provides science-based advice to promote health and to reduce risk for major chronic diseases through diet and physical activity. Major causes of morbidity and mortality [meaning illness and death] in the United States are related to poor diet and a sedentary lifestyle."

Even the World Health Organization finds the impact of diet on the prevalence of chronic disease to be an issue of global importance. According to the World Health Organization's 2003 report titled *Global Strategy on Diet, Physical Activity and Health*:

- Up to 2.7 million lives could be saved annually with sufficient fruit and vegetable consumption.
- Low fruit and vegetable intake is among the top ten selected risk factors for global mortality.
- Worldwide, low intake of fruits and vegetables is estimated to cause about 19 percent of all gastrointestinal cancer cases, 31 percent of all ischemic heart disease cases, and 11 percent of stroke cases.

The Old Food Pyramid

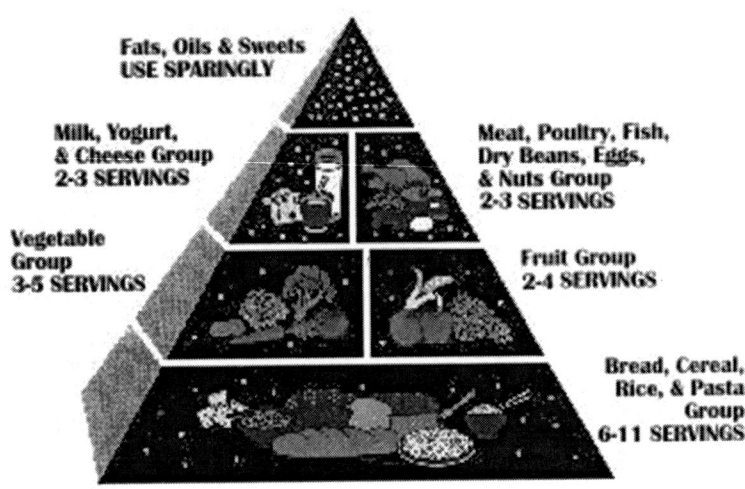

The old food pyramid made no distinction between high-fat and low-fat dairy products, lumping milk and cheese together. And as the USDA continues to do, the old pyramid grouped "dry beans" and marbled red meat together in the same category. Somehow, lumping plant-based, nutrient-rich legumes and monounsaturated fat-laden nuts together with highly saturated red meat in the same food category flies in the face of common sense. Even more humorous, candy and other nonnutritive snacks were positioned at the pinnacle of the pyramid—like a metaphorical star on a Christmas tree.

The New Food Pyramid

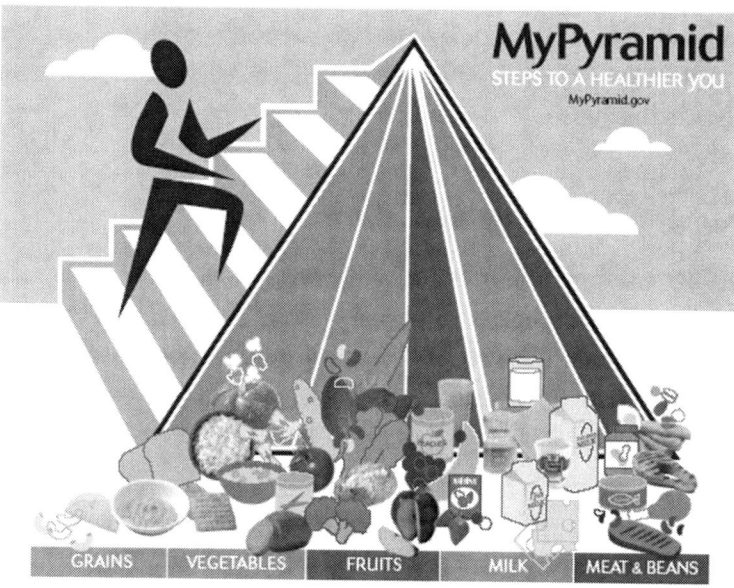

The new food pyramid made huge strides in incorporating some key themes, including the following:

- Activity goals.
- Age-, gender-, and activity-based calorie needs.
- Proportionality (colored bands indicating amounts from each food group).
- Acknowledges important concepts such as *trans* fats, whole grains, and the introduction of "discretionary calories"—a term used to indicate the amount of nonnutritive calories one might consume and still be healthy.

Still, the dietary guidelines continue to exist without addressing timely concerns such as genetically modified organisms (GMO's), organic foods, food additives, and sugar substitutes.

Activity

Most Americans would be astounded to learn that scientific experts recommend sixty minutes of daily exercise for those trying to manage their weight. For those trying to lose weight, the guideline is ninety minutes of daily physical activity.

Recommended Energy or Calorie Needs

By accessing www.mypyramid.gov, you can estimate your energy needs by entering your gender, age, and activity level. Interestingly, the needs for most women average 1,200–1,600 calories, and for most men 1,800–2,500 calories. However, the current food labels use 2,000- and 2,500-calorie intakes as a reference point.

* Percent Daily Values are based on a 2,000 calorie diet. Your Daily Values may be higher or lower depending on your calorie needs.

	Calories:	2,000	2,500
Total Fat	Less than	65g	80g
Sat Fat	Less than	20g	25g
Cholesterol	Less than	300mg	300mg
Sodium	Less than	2,400mg	2,400mg
Total Carbohydrate		300g	375g
Dietary Fiber		25g	30g

Proportionality: Amounts from Each Food Group Defined

GRAINS Make half your grains whole	VEGETABLES Vary your veggies	FRUITS Focus on fruits	MILK Get your calcium-rich foods	MEAT & BEANS Go lean with protein
Eat at least 3 oz. of whole-grain cereals, breads, crackers, rice, or pasta every day 1 oz. is about 1 slice of bread, about 1 cup of breakfast cereal, or ½ cup of cooked rice, cereal, or pasta	Eat more dark-green veggies like broccoli, spinach, and other dark leafy greens Eat more orange vegetables like carrots and sweetpotatoes Eat more dry beans and peas like pinto beans, kidney beans, and lentils	Eat a variety of fruit Choose fresh, frozen, canned, or dried fruit Go easy on fruit juices	Go low-fat or fat-free when you choose milk, yogurt, and other milk products If you don't or can't consume milk, choose lactose-free products or other calcium sources such as fortified foods and beverages	Choose low-fat or lean meats and poultry Bake it, broil it, or grill it Vary your protein routine — choose more fish, beans, peas, nuts, and seeds
For a 2,000-calorie diet, you need the amounts below from each food group. To find the amounts that are right for you, go to MyPyramid.gov.				
Eat 6 oz. every day	Eat 2½ cups every day	Eat 2 cups every day	Get 3 cups every day; for kids aged 2 to 8, it's 2	Eat 5½ oz. every day

Source: www.mypyramid.gov

The colored bands in the new food pyramid suggest the proportion of our diets that each food group should make up.

Serving sizes are defined in the following way:[1]

- The **Fruit Group** includes all fresh, frozen, canned, and dried fruits and fruit juices. In general, one cup of fruit or 100 percent fruit juice, or one-half cup of dried fruit can be considered as one cup from the fruit group.
- The **Vegetable Group** includes all fresh, frozen, canned, and dried vegetables and vegetable juices. In general, one cup of raw or cooked vegetables or vegetable juice, or two cups of raw leafy greens can be considered as one cup from the vegetable group.
- The **Grains Group** includes all foods made from wheat, rice, oats, cornmeal, and barley, such as bread, pasta, oatmeal, breakfast cereals, tortillas, and grits. In general, one slice of bread, one cup of ready-to-eat cereal, or one-half cup of cooked rice, pasta, or cooked

---

1 (http://www.mypyramid.gov/downloads/MyPyramid_Food_Intake_Patterns.pdf)

cereal can be considered as one ounce from the grains group. *At least half of all grains consumed should be whole grains.*

Of note, it was finally recommended by the USDA that at *least* half of all grains and starches consumed be "whole grain." This is actually easier said than done, as current labeling practices make it difficult to determine what "whole grain" actually is.

For example, "made with whole grain" means the food may be made with a lot or a little whole grain. "Multigrain" means the food is made with a mixture, but it could still be mostly refined flour. "100 percent whole grain" means made with no refined flour, while "whole grain" means that at least 51 percent of the product is whole grain. A label that states that the product is "100 percent whole grain" is the best choice when looking for whole-grain products. The next best choice is one where the first ingredient says "whole grain."

- In the **Meat and Beans Group,** one ounce of lean meat, poultry, or fish; one egg; one tablespoon peanut butter; one-fourth cup cooked legumes (kidney, pinto, chickpeas, and so on); or one-half ounce of nuts or seeds can generally be considered a one ounce-equivalent.
- The **Milk Group** includes all milk products and foods made from milk, such as yogurt and cheese. Foods made from milk that have little to no calcium, such as cream cheese, cream, and butter, are not part of the group. Most milk group choices should be fat-free or low-fat. In general, one cup of milk or yogurt, one and a half ounces of natural cheese, or two ounces of processed cheese can be considered as one cup from the milk group.
- **Oils** include fats such as canola, corn, olive, soybean, and sunflower oils. Some foods are naturally high in oils, such as nuts, olives, some fish, and avocados. Foods that are mainly oil include mayonnaise, certain salad dressings, and soft margarine.

At long last, the dietary recommendations finally indicated that there is *no* dietary need for *trans* fats—the form of fat created from hydrogenating or hardening liquid vegetable oil, which increases shelf life but adversely becomes artery clogging as a result. In fact, we should avoid *trans* fats altogether.

The Harvard School of Public Health Food Pyramid

The Harvard School of Public Health food pyramid developed by Dr. Walt Willet in his book *Eat, Drink and Be Healthy* Free Press/Simon & Schuster, Inc. 2005 is probably the best food guide for most Americans eating a traditional western-style diet. Here there is no pretense that meat and beans are nutritionally equivalent. In fact, red meat and butter are right up there with refined processed food as items we should eat sparingly. In addition, healthy vegetable oils are separated out as something to eat frequently, not to be limited. Although controversial, Walt Willett also suggests that dairy products need to be consumed only twice a day, if at all, as opposed to the USDA guidelines that recommends three servings daily.

The DASH Food Pyramid

The Dietary Approaches to Stop Hypertension (DASH) diet developed by the National Institutes of Health and the National Heart Lung and Blood Institute has demonstrated the ability to use diet to lower blood pressure—in many cases equivalent to the same response people have to blood pressure medications. A blood pressure drop of just a few points can reduce the chances of having a heart attack or stroke. *(http://www.nhlbi. nih.gov/health/public/heart/hbp/dash/new_dash.pdf)*

Despite the subtle variations in these food pyramids, one consistent message remains unchallenged: we need to eat *more* fruits and vegetables!

Variety with Fruits and Vegetables

Variety in your diet gives you the greatest chance of obtaining a range of nutrients. Including a range of fruits and vegetables assures you access to the tens of thousands of yet uncategorized phytochemicals—compounds found in plant foods that offer innumerable benefits in an exciting new area of scientific research.

With the ever-changing nutritional messages and evolving scientific research, it can be difficult to draw steadfast conclusions. However, one message has always been consistent: fruits and vegetables are good for you! And yet, we do not seem to get the message. The majority of Americans do not achieve the recommended goal of five or more servings of fruits and vegetables daily. In fact, only one in four of us routinely achieve this goal, according to *Trends in Fruit and Vegetable Consumption among Adults in the United States: Behavioral Risk Factor Surveillance System, 1994–2000*. Five or more servings of fruits and vegetables may sound overwhelming, but let's review a sample daily menu:

- Breakfast: three-fourths cup of orange juice with cereal
- Midmorning snack: Fruit included
- Lunch: one cup of vegetable soup or a large salad with meal
- Dinner: one cup of your favorite cooked vegetable included with meal
- Evening: snack on a piece of fruit

That's seven servings of fruits and vegetables!

In fact, the traditional "five-a-day" program referring to the number of fruits and vegetables we should eat daily—is now the "seven-to-nine-a-day" program!

Current USDA dietary guidelines suggest:

- nine servings of fruits and vegetables a day for men and active teens
- seven servings of fruits and vegetables a day for women and kids ages seven and up
- five servings of fruits and vegetables a day for children ages two to six

What does this mean?

For example, let's say a household is made up of two adults and two small children. Assuming that all servings of fruits and vegetables were prepared at home (which is a pretty safe bet in my family, anyway), the grocery cart from the weekly shopping would need to contain about two hundred servings of fruits and vegetables per week!

- Man: 9 svgs daily x 7 days = 63
- Woman: 7 svgs daily x 7 days = 49
- Child aged 7: 7 svgs daily x 7 days = 49
- Child aged 5: 5 svgs daily x 7 days = 35

The first time I actually went to the grocery store intent on selecting the amount of fruits and vegetables I would need to meet this guideline for the week, I had little room in the cart for much else. When I returned home from grocery shopping, the first question my husband asked was, "Where are my snack foods?" I explained that I had no room for them after purchasing so many fresh fruits and vegetables, and I think that is exactly the point.

How are we doing?

According to the CDC's National Health and Nutrition Examination Survey:

- Only 12 percent of children from ages two to eighteen are considered to have a diet that meets dietary guidelines
- Only one in every five individuals met the dietary recommendation during 1994–96.
- 40 percent of household meal planners/preparers are dietary optimists—that is, they rate their diet quality to be better than it actually is. The same proportion are dietary realists—they accurately rate their diet quality. The remaining 20 percent are dietary pessimists—they perceive their diet quality to be worse than it actually is.

Evaluate: How am I really doing?

Truly, the only way to really know how well you are doing is to write your food intake down.

The following worksheet provided by the USDA (My Pyramid Worksheet from www.mypyramid.gov) provides an easy way to determine how well your diet stacks up against the recommendations. Try it for a couple days and see how you do.

Write in Your Choices for Today	Food Group	Tip	Goal	List each food choice in its food group	Estimate Your Total
	GRAINS	Make at least half your grains whole grains	6 ounce equivalents (1 ounce equivalent is about 1 slice bread, 1 cup dry cereal, or ½ cup rice or pasta)		ounce equivalents
	VEGETABLES	Try to have vegetables from several subgroups each day	2 ½ cups Subgroups: Dark Green, Orange, Starchy, Dry Beans and Peas, Other Veggies		cups
	FRUITS	Make most choices fruit, not juice	2 cups		cups
	MILK	Choose fat-free or low fat most often	3 cups (1 ½ ounces cheese = 1 cup milk)		cups
	MEAT & BEANS	Choose lean meat and poultry. Vary your choices—more fish, beans, peas, nuts, and seeds	5 ½ ounce equivalents (1 ounce equivalent is 1 ounce meat, poultry or fish, 1 T. peanut butter, ½ ounce nuts, ¼ cup dry beans or peas)		ounce equivalents
	PHYSICAL ACTIVITY	Build more physical activity into your daily routine at home and work.	At least 30 minutes of moderate to vigorous activity a day. 10 minutes or more at a time.	*Some foods don't fit into any group. These "extras" may be mainly fat or sugar—limit your intake of these.	minutes

How did you do today? ☐ Great ☐ So-So ☐ Not so Great

My food goal for tomorrow is:

My activity goal for tomorrow is:

Tradeoffs: Convenience versus Cost

One can make a healthy choice that is time efficient or convenient *or* one that is economical. It comes down to personal choice. Often we must choose between convenience and cost and make the best choice for us as individuals and our families. Here are two examples:

Smoothie:
- Brand name: three dollars per bottle
- Homemade: pennies each

Fruit Popsicle:
- Brand name: more than three dollars per package
- Homemade: pennies each

Either is a good choice; what matters is that you make the choice that is best for you.

Tips for Incorporating the Food Pyramid Guidelines into Your Diet

- Make change gradually, but have a goal in mind.
- Remember that your shopping cart contents should reflect what is ultimately served on the plate.
- Your kitchen cabinets, refrigerator, and freezer should also reflect the same breakdown as the food pyramid.
- Plan your meals ahead as much as possible.

- Breakfast:
    o Add dried fruit or fresh fruit to cereal.
    o Drink a variety of juices.

- Snacks:
    - Create a beautiful snack plate with raw fruit and vegetable options. Use yogurt, salad dressing, or hummus for a dip.
    - Make your own snack packs of dried fruit and granola for the car.

- Lunch:
    - Make sure there's juice in that juice box!
    - Use colorful, appealing containers.
    - Let your kids make some choices.
    - Try to include a fruit and vegetable as often as possible.

- Dinner:
    - Increase variety
    - Use fresh ingredients.
    - Add creativity by trying new recipes.
    - Commit to serving new foods multiple times. It is a necessary requirement before a picky eater will try them.

The Food Pyramid Simplified

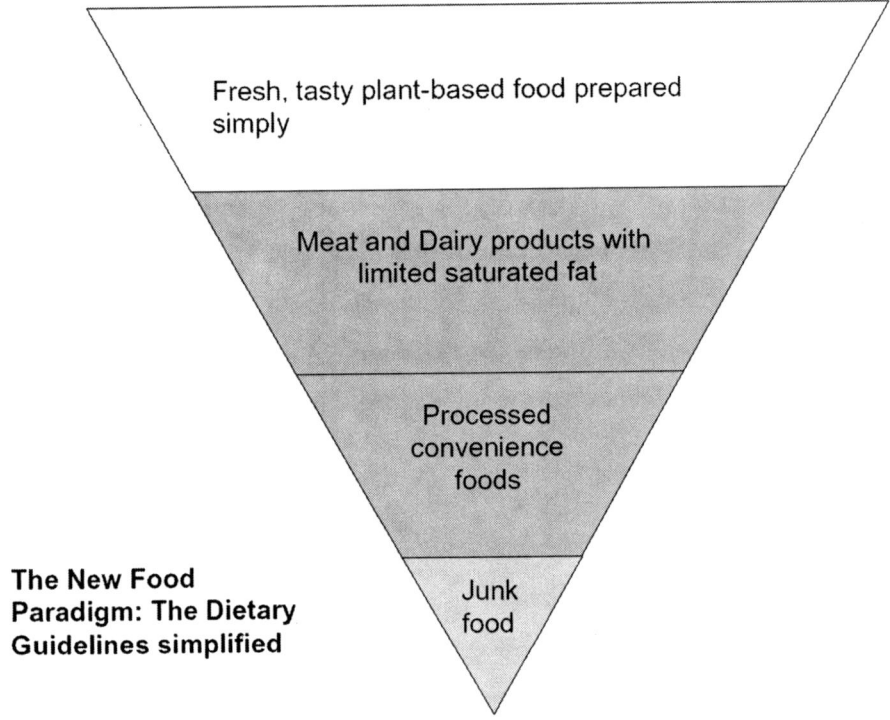

This is our attempt to come up with a simple food pyramid anybody can follow. We upturned the pyramid on its head, and find that it distills all of the scientific research into its simplest form.

Summary Recommendations: The Dietary Guidelines Simplified

- Show respect for your body and the Earth.
- Experience joy when eating, especially with friends and family.
- Food is not just a collection of nutrients—it defines your ethnicity, heritage, health, preferences, and values. Choose wisely.
- Eat a variety of fresh, tasty, plant-based foods prepared simply.

Take Action

- Access the USDA food pyramid Web site (www.pyramid.gov). Print your personal food intake guidelines.
- Use the worksheet included in this chapter to keep your own food record.
- Evaluate how well you are meeting the food pyramid guidelines.
- If your kids are old enough, have them participate as well. Post your food records on the refrigerator and compare.

Chapter 6:
Grocery Shopping Guidelines

He that won't be counseled can't be helped.
—Benjamin Franklin

It has been my observation that people are just about as happy as they make up their mind to be.
—Abraham Lincoln

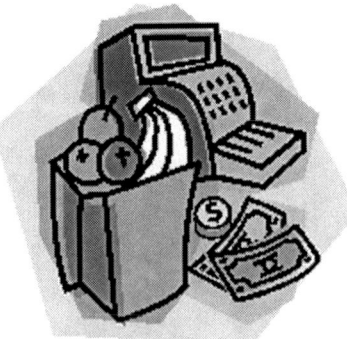

> Objective:
> - How can make healthier choices when shopping for groceries?
> - How can I incorporate menu planning and grocery lists into my shopping routine?

Eating a healthy diet requires advance planning. If you don't have the right ingredients in the home to make healthy meals, it is easy to resort to dining out. Busy lifestyles with children in extracurricular activities, often occurring at the dinner hour, make organizing a meal challenging *without* prior planning. Actually, just keeping ahead of the laundry can make our lives very busy!

Where do you start? First, ask yourself, your children, or spouse, "What do you want for breakfast, lunch and dinner this week?" By involving others in the meal planning, you not only ensure they will enjoy meals, but also take off some of the pressure of planning all of the meals yourself. When you have several breakfast, lunch, and dinner menus written down, start a grocery list. Simply put your menus on the left side of the list and all the ingredients needed on the right side.

Shop on the edge. Shop on the grocery store's edge, that is. The perimeter is the place where the healthiest foods are found—produce, fresh meats, dairy, fresh seafood, and fresh baked goods. The center aisles typically contain snack foods, processed foods, frozen foods, cereals, and so on. They still contain some healthy choices, but those are the exception, not the rule.

Choose foods in their simplest form with the least amount of packaging. This guideline will lead you to the healthiest foods with a minimum of label reading. Best of all, if you don't buy prepackaged or microwaveable processed foods, your kids won't eat them and you won't either!

Discretion in your calories. The USDA dietary guidelines call "discretionary calories" the two hundred calories left after you have consumed all of the healthy foods in your day. Unfortunately, two hundred calories won't get you very far. This would be equivalent to one soda or sweet beverage, one candy bar (maybe), one serving of chips, or one half-cup cup of decadent ice cream.

If your grocery cart for the week contains only two hundred discretionary calories per person in your household (assuming everybody is eating only healthy foods throughout the day away from home and no one is trying to lose weight), this would leave little room in the cart for extras. A large bag of chips and a half gallon of ice cream would be about it for a family of four.

Whatever your family size, limit the number of snack foods you will make available at one time in your home. For example, each child gets to choose one snack item for the week.

Buy what you enjoy eating, but make your own limits. Is there something you tend to eat too much of or isn't good for you? If you must have a bowl of ice cream every night, at least consider buying the smallest portion size possible. You might buy Hershey's Kisses instead of the big chocolate bar, individual-sized bags of chips instead of the bargain bag, or the tiny four-ounce cans of soda instead of the two-liter bottles. Bulk quantities that are on sale may be cheaper on the wallet, but not to your body.

Try something new each time. Each time you go grocery shopping, try to put something new on your shopping cart that you have not tried before. This will automatically add more variety, increase your awareness of new foods, make grocery shopping more fun, and maybe even lead to the discovery of a new favorite. Sometimes you may find something you don't like and will never buy again. Consider it an important part of discovery, and keep trying new things!

Eat with color. A daily palette of fruits and vegetables that include the colors red, yellow/orange, green, blue/purple, and white will ensure that you get all of the micronutrients you and your family need for optimal health. Colorful fruits and vegetables provide the wide range of vitamins, minerals, fiber, and phytochemicals your body uses to maintain good health and energy levels, protect against the effects of aging, and reduce the risk of cancer and heart disease when part of a low fat diet.

Many of the phytochemicals and other compounds that make fruits and vegetables good for us also give them their color. That's why it's essential to sample the complete color spectrum every day to get the full preventive benefits of fruits and vegetables.

- o Blue/purple fruits and vegetables contain varying amounts of health-promoting phytochemicals, such as **anthocyanins** and **phenolics**, currently being studied for their antioxidant and anti-aging benefits.
- o Green vegetables contain varying amounts of phytochemicals such as **lutein** and **indoles**, which interest researchers because of their potential antioxidant, health-promoting benefits.
- o White, tan, and brown fruits and vegetables contain varying amounts of phytochemicals of interest to scientists. These include **allicin**, found in the garlic and onion family. The mineral **selenium**, found in mushrooms, is also the subject of research.
- o Yellow and orange fruits and vegetables contain varying amounts of antioxidants such as **vitamin C**, as well as **carotenoids** and **bioflavonoids**, two classes of phytochemicals that scientists are studying for their health-promoting potential.
- o Specific phytochemicals in the red group that are being studied for their health-promoting properties include **lycopene** and **anthocyanins**.

Include the following in your grocery shopping to ensure you and your family are 'eating with color.'

- Fresh fruits and vegetables of any kind
- Frozen fruits and vegetables without added sauces or added fat and sodium
- Dried fruits or vegetables
- Canned fruits packed in juice only

- Canned vegetables with attention paid to sodium content (less than three hundred milligrams per serving)
- Jarred tomato sauce
- Salsas
- Vegetable juice with attention to sodium content
- Fruit juice: 100 percent without any additives
- Unsweetened applesauce and other fruit sauces
- Unsweetened preserves or spreadable fruit
- Fruit sorbets and smoothies (watch the sugar content)

Add whole grains to your grocery list. There are many varieties of whole grains to choose from, including rice (of which there are also many different varieties), kashi, quinoa, amaranth, bulgur, barley, millet, wheat berries, oats, spelt, couscous, corn grits or cornmeal, and whole grain bread.

Oat bran contains soluble fiber, which may lower cholesterol levels. It can be substituted in recipes that call for flour. You can also add it to muffin and quick bread recipes, or use it as a coating on seafood or poultry.

Wheat germ is an excellent source of vitamin E. Add it to quick bread and muffin recipes or pancake batter. You might also simply sprinkle it over your favorite hot breakfast cereal or over yogurt.

Wheat bran or unprocessed bran can be sprinkled over cereal. It is high in fiber. Limit your serving size to one to two tablespoons.

Cracked wheat is wheat berries cracked into small pieces. Cook using one cup grain to two cups fluid, and use it in tabbouleh salad and side grain dishes.

Pearl barley can be cooked with 1 cup grain to 3 1/2 cups fluid. Pearl barley tastes great in soups, stews, and rice pilafs. It is also nice in cold salad with feta cheese and cucumbers, similar to tabbouleh salad.

Quinoa is a light, nutty-flavored grain. It tends to expand to four times its size when cooked. Use quinoa in salads, stuffed tomatoes, and other side dishes. Cook with one cup grain to two cups fluid.

Spelt is also a light, nutty-flavored grain. It's rich in magnesium and B vitamins and higher in protein than wheat. Spelt is tasty in pilafs and salads. The grain-to-liquid ratio should be one cup grain: three cups spelt berries.

Buckwheat groats (kasha) are not part of the wheat family. Cook with one cup grain: two cups fluid.

Bulgur is cracked wheat that has been partially cooked. Cook using 1 cup grain to 2 1/2 cups fluid.

Choose cereals or breads with two or more grams of fiber.

- Try whole-grain pasta or at least a whole-wheat blend such as *Ronzoni Healthy Harvest.*
- Choose converted or slow-cooking brown rice. Avoid instant white rice.
- Try barley in rice pilaf mixtures.
- Make side dishes with quinoa, wheat berries or other different whole grains (see recipe).

Add noncaloric beverages to your grocery list such as:

- Seltzers without added sweeteners
- Sparkling waters
- Spring waters
- Flavored waters without added sweeteners
- Unsweetened teas
- Coffee in moderation without high-fat additives such as cream, whole milk, nondairy creamer

Add low fat protein sources to your grocery list. Both meat and dairy products contain saturated fat. Since twenty grams of both saturated and *trans* fats are considered an upper limit, even low-fat dairy products and meats need to be consumed in moderation.

Many delicious, brand-name cheeses come in lower fat alternatives, *including Cabot, Kraft's Cracker Barrel, Alpine Lace,* and *Healthy Choice.* Skim milk is best, but if you aren't used to it, start with 2 percent milk and then switch to 1 percent. Ultimately, you will get used to skim milk for many uses. Soy milk is also a good choice.

- Low-fat meats (less than five grams saturated fat per four-ounce cooked serving)
    - Turkey breast
    - Lean ground turkey breast
    - Lean ground chicken breast
    - Chicken breast
    - Turkey leg
    - Veal leg, top round
    - Beef eye of the round, top round, or bottom round (select)
    - Chicken drumstick
    - Pork tenderloin
    - Veal shoulder
    - Lamb shank
    - Beef top round (choice)
    - Veal shoulder, blade
    - Beef tip round (choice)
    - Pork top loin
    - Ham, leg, rump half
    - Pork center loin

- Pork sirloin
- Beef top sirloin (select)
- Chicken thigh
- Lamb sirloin

Some low fat meat substitutions to consider when grocery shopping include the following:

If you eat:	Try this:
Bacon	Turkey bacon
Salami	Turkey salami
Pastrami	Turkey pastrami (in the deli section of the grocery store)
Meatballs	Meatballs made from ground turkey. Look for ready-made meatballs in the freezer section of your grocery store.
Hot dogs	Low-fat hot dogs with less than five grams of fat per hot dog
Hamburgers	-Try ground turkey, or mix lean ground beef with ground turkey. -Try ground buffalo meat, which is available in some grocery stores. -Try meatless hamburgers like the *Morningstar Farms* brand, but be sure to add lots of condiments!
Meatloaf	Make with ground turkey rather than ground beef.
Sausage	Turkey sausage (many different varieties available)
Breakfast sausage	*Morningstar Farms* vegetarian breakfast sausage links

Add fish to your grocery list.

Fish can be a very healthy protein source, with the added benefit of containing heart-healthy fatty acids. Populations that eat a lot of fish (such as those in Sweden and Norway) have a lower incidence of strokes and heart disease. Current American Heart Association dietary guidelines suggest eating fish two times per week.

Unfortunately, nearly all fish and shellfish today contain traces of mercury. Mercury has found its way into our fish supply due to industrial pollution. For most people (unless you are an Inuit Eskimo, where severe learning disabilities have been attributed to high levels of mercury in seal and fish consumed there), the risk from mercury by eating fish and shellfish is not a serious health concern—at least not as serious as heart disease, which is the number one killer in the United States and whose risk can be significantly reduced through diet and exercise.

However, some fish and shellfish contain higher levels of mercury that may harm an unborn baby or young child's developing nervous system. The risks from mercury in fish and shellfish depend on the amount of fish and shellfish eaten and the levels of mercury contained in them. The Food and Drug Administration (FDA) and the Environmental Protection Agency (EPA) have suggestions for limiting the amount and kinds of fish pregnant women and young children should consume.

U.S. Food and Drug Administration Advisory: What You Need to Know about Mercury in Fish and Shellfish (2004):

For:
Women Who Might Become Pregnant
Women Who Are Pregnant
Nursing Mothers
Young Children

By following these three recommendations for selecting and eating fish or shellfish, women and young children will receive the benefits of eating fish and shellfish and be confident that they have reduced their exposure to the harmful effects of mercury.

1. Do not eat shark, swordfish, king mackerel, or tilefish because they contain high levels of mercury.
2. Eat up to twelve ounces (two average meals) a week of a variety of fish and shellfish that are lower in mercury.
    o Five of the most commonly eaten fish that are low in mercury are shrimp, canned light tuna, salmon, pollock, and catfish.
    o Another commonly eaten fish, albacore ("white") tuna has more mercury than canned light tuna. So, when choosing your two meals of fish and shellfish, you may eat up to six ounces (one average meal) of albacore tuna per week.
3. Check local advisories about the safety of fish caught by family and friends in your local lakes, rivers, and coastal areas. If no advice is available, eat up to six ounces (one average meal) per week of fish you catch from local waters, but don't consume any other fish during that week.

Follow these same recommendations when feeding fish and shellfish to your young child, but serve smaller portions.

Source: http://www.fda.gov/bbs/topics/news/2004/NEW01038.html

Add other low fat protein sources to your grocery list such as the following:

Eggs. Nowadays eggs come in all varieties—fresh, natural, organic, free range, cage-free, no antibiotics, fed vegetarian diet, contains omega-3 fatty acids, small farm raised—and are certified by a variety of different third parties. The definitions of these parameters (except for the term "organic") vary as well. At this time, these labels are ill defined for eggs.

Peas, beans, legumes, and lentils—dry or canned. There are many to experiment with, including soybeans, pinto beans, chickpeas, lentils (red, green, and yellow), cranberry beans, black-eyed peas, pink beans, navy beans, black beans, whole beans, lima beans, kidney beans, great northern beans, adzuki beans, mung beans, fava beans, and more.

Soy products. Soy products come in many textures,. Brands such as *Morningstar Farms* and *Boca* make a variety of soy-based products that you might want to try, including burgers, chicken-like nuggets, breakfast sausage links, and meatballs.

Other items to add to your grocery list include:

- Nuts: preferably unroasted and without salt
- Nut butters: all-natural peanut butter made from 100 percent peanuts, other nut butters are also available (such as almond butter and cashew butter)
- Seeds: preferably unroasted and without salt
- Vegetable oils: preferably canola, olive, grapeseed, or nut oils, flavored oils
- Salad dressings: preferably made with olive, grapeseed, or canola oil
- Mayonnaise: preferably made with canola oil

Choose the following sparingly when grocery shopping:

- Full-fat dairy products such as whole milk, high-fat ice cream, and frozen desserts
- Packaged, processed foods
- Fatty cuts of meat

- Deli or processed meats such as hot dogs, bacon, or sausage
- Foods sweetened with sugar
- Sweet desserts of all kinds
- Foods with more than three hundred milligrams of sodium per serving

---

A Word about Snacks

So your kid only eats chocolate cookies one after the other right out of the bag and never stops? Goes right to the cabinet for the whole jumbo bag of chips and then eats them in one sitting? Here are some suggestions for warding off the junk food binges:

> **Chocolate chip cookie kid.** Buy frozen chocolate chip cookie dough. Make only a few cookies at a time, but satisfy the craving. Make your own chocolate chip cookie dough (see the recipe for oatmeal chocolate chip cookies), and keep it in the freezer. Slice off and bake a few at a time. This is less expensive and can be healthier.
>
> **Chip kid.** Look for healthier snack alternatives: low-fat tortilla chips, baked potato chips, and low-fat popcorn. Make your own popcorn on the stove. Buy only single serving size bags—not jumbo bags of chips.
>
> **Ice cream kid.** Bring ice cream out only as a special treat, and keep a healthier frozen dessert alternative on hand like low-fat fudgsicles or popsicles. Buy small, kid-size ice cream cups, or even better, individual popsicles made with 100 percent juice.

Suggestions for Snacks

Don't view snacks as a digression from healthy eating at mealtimes. Instead, look at them as an opportunity to keep you or your kids from getting so hungry that you or they can't make a healthy choice. A snack is an opportunity to add even more nutrition to your day, and if done right, can give you an energy boost. Here are some healthy suggestions:

- Multigrain crackers made without hydrogenated vegetable or partially hydrogenated vegetable oils (also known as trans fats) with peanut butter
- Trail mixes made with nuts and fruit with a glass of low-fat milk
- Tortilla chips with a salsa or a black bean dip
- Bread sticks with hummus or baba ganoush (a Middle Eastern spread made with eggplant)
- Rice cakes with a fruit spread
- Low-fat popcorn
- Pretzel sticks and low-fat cheese dip
- Pita crisps
- Unsweetened applesauce cups
- Carrots with a low-fat dressing dip
- Whole-grain bagel with low-fat cream cheese
- Apple slices with walnuts
- Canned fruit with yogurt and granola topping

For Baking

For those who bake at home or want to begin baking at home, here is a core list of ingredients to have on hand to make the recipes in this book.

- Wheat germ
- Flaxseed (ground)

- White whole-wheat flour—a particular variety of wheat flour which is whiter in appearance than traditional wheat flour milled from darker varieties
- Baking powder
- Baking soda
- Cornmeal
- Eggs
- Canola oil
- Vanilla
- Spices: cinnamon, ginger, cloves, cumin, chili powder, thyme, sage, and others

Condiments. These are the essentials that turn food from good to great. Some condiments to include in your kitchen area ground pepper mill, kosher salt, sea salt, low-salt soy sauce, mustard, chili sauce, hot sauces, Worcestershire sauce, vinegar, honey, salsas, fresh herbs such as parsley and scallions, and fresh ginger root (keep in the freezer to keep it fresh).

Take Action

Using the recommendations above, make a weekly menu plan and highlight what you plan to buy on your next trip to the grocery store. Add to it as needed, and delete what you don't need. Use it as a reference tool to begin menu planning for making your family the healthiest, most delicious meals possible. Focus on colors. Make sure to consider your kids' preferences and include one of their favorite meals and snacks. The art of menu planning has gone by the wayside of "wash day" and "market day." In the name of good nutrition, it needs to be rediscovered! Even if you have never done this before, try it this week. Use the following worksheet to create your menus for the week. Make sure you have all of the ingredients on hand to bring your menus to life.

DINNER	Protein source	Vegetable	Starch	Salad	Dessert/Fruit	Other
Sunday						
Monday						
Tuesday						
Wednesday						
Thursday						
Friday						
Saturday						

BREAKFAST	Fruit	Starch	Beverage	Other
Sunday				
Monday				
Tuesday				
Wednesday				
Thursday				
Friday				
Saturday				

LUNCH	Protein source	Vegetable	Starch	Salad	Dessert/Fruit	Other
Sunday						
Monday						
Tuesday						
Wednesday						
Thursday						
Friday						
Saturday						

Chapter 7:

Eating on the Run: It's All in the Planning!

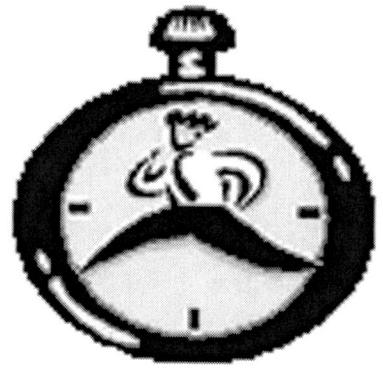

"The welfare of the family, both physical and spiritual, is largely in the hands of the one who provides the 'three meals a day.'"
—Mary Swartz Rose, *Feeding the Family*

Objectives:
- If I'm on the run, what choices can I make to pursue good nutrition for me and my family?
- How can I ensure that my children eat a healthy lunch at school?
- How can I prepare the ultimate brown bag lunch?

Skipping to Breakfast. Feeding your family a healthy breakfast can be a daunting task, as this is often the busiest time of the day for many of us. If you have discussed breakfast preferences with your family in advance, preparing breakfast will be a whole lot easier. Depending on the age of your children and their culinary abilities, try to incorporate their talents into the meal preparation. Breakfast is essential to get your body going after an evening of rest. It is hard to get the mind going without food. If your child is not a big breakfast eater, try to get him or her to eat a smaller portion. Good nutritional habits begin at home. Be a healthy role model for your child!

At breakfast time, try to incorporate some energy-boosting foods such as oatmeal, whole-grain cereal, whole-grain breads, English muffins, whole-grain granola bars, or a whole grain coupled with a good source of protein such as milk, yogurt, cheese, and peanut butter. *Kashi* brand granola bars are also a great source of carbohydrates (energy food) and protein; try these when you need a quick fix.

Of additional importance is the body's need for hydration in the morning. This is an important habit for children who may not get a beverage until they have a midmorning snack or lunch. Remember that the body has been without fluids for eight to ten hours during sleep. So don't forget to replenish with water. Try to enjoy a healthy breakfast as a family; if not during the work week, then try for a family breakfast on the weekend.

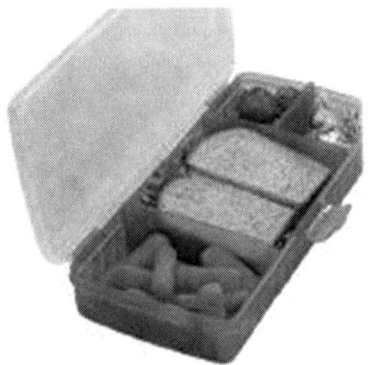

Joining the Lunch Bunch: Make an "UnLunchable. "Buying lunch at school may be the first time your child gets to call the shots about which foods he or she will eat. The good news is that school lunches have improved over the years, both in taste and nutrition. Some schools also have made an effort to serve better dishes, such as grilled chicken sandwiches and salads. Unfortunately, although many school lunches meet the standards for protein, vitamins, calcium, and iron, they still exceed recommendations for fat.

School lunches are improving, but not as much as many nutritionists and parents would hope. As we continue to push for healthier lunch options in the schools—and this requires a partnership among parents, the school, and the government—let's try to have our children make, or at least take, a healthy, tasty lunch from home.

Making lunch does not have to be difficult. Use school lunches to steer your child toward good choices. Together you and your child can come up with favorite brown bag lunches, making it easier to eat healthy. Here are some other steps to take:

Look over the cafeteria menu with your child. Ask what a typical lunch includes and which meals he or she particularly likes. Recommend items that are healthier, but be willing to allow your child to buy favorite lunch items occasionally, even if that includes a hot dog. After all, moderation is the key.

- Ask about foods such as chips, soda, and ice cream. Find out if and when these foods are available at school.
- Encourage your child to pack a lunch, at least occasionally. If you do it right, this can put you back in the driver's seat and help you ensure that your child is getting a nutritious midday meal.

Healthier Alternatives

Encourage your child to choose cafeteria meals that include fruits, vegetables, lean meats, and whole grains, such as wheat bread instead of white.

Also, suggest that they avoid fried foods when possible and choose low-fat milk or water as a drink.

If you're helping your child pack a lunch, start by brainstorming foods and snacks that he or she would like to eat. In addition to old standbys, such as peanut butter and jelly, try pitas or wrap sandwiches stuffed with grilled chicken or veggies. Try soups and salads, if your child is willing, and don't forget last night's leftovers as an easy lunchbox filler.

You also can take your child's current lunch and perform a lunch makeover. Here are some suggestions for small changes that make a nutritional difference.

Instead of:	Consider:
Higher-fat lunch meats (bologna, salami)	Lower-fat deli meats (turkey)
White bread	Whole-grain breads (wheat, oat, multigrain)
Mayonnaise	Light mayonnaise or mustard
Fried chips and snacks	Baked chips, air-popped popcorn, trail mix, veggies and dip
Fruit in syrup	Fruit in natural juices or fresh fruit
Cookies and snack cakes	Trail mix, yogurt, or homemade baked goods such as oatmeal cookies or fruit muffins
Fruit drinks and soda	Milk, water, or 100% fruit juice

To ensure a balanced lunch, try to incorporate a variety of healthy ingredients.

Making the Ultimate Brown-Bag Lunch

1. Choose a **carbohydrate**. Use whole grains as a side with a salad, or use to make a sandwich.

- Mini whole-wheat pita pocket
- Oatmeal bread
- Multigrain bread
- Whole-grain wrap
- Side of brown rice
- Side of whole-wheat pasta

2. Add your **veggies**. Top a sandwich or make a salad with:

- Lettuce
- Tomato
- Shredded carrot
- Broccoli slaw
- Sprouts
- Roasted pepper
- Cherry tomatoes
- Baby carrots

3. Add a **protein** source to your sandwich or top your salad with it:

- Tuna (limit to one time a week, due to high mercury levels)
- Turkey slices
- Grilled chicken
- Reduced-fat grated cheese
- Hummus
- Sliced eggs

- Black beans, kidney beans, or chickpeas

4. Add a side:

- Light popcorn
- Flavored mini rice cakes
- Reduced-fat, whole-grain crackers such as Wheat Thins or reduced-fat Triscuits
- Pretzels
- Low-fat granola bar
- Yogurt

5. Don't forget the **fruit:**

- Fifteen grapes
- One small banana
- One cup strawberries
- One small apple or pear (if cutting, toss with fresh lemon juice to prevent browning)
- Kiwi (cut in half and serve with a spoon; the fruit can be scooped out)
- Two tablespoons raisins or other dried fruit

6. Add a **beverage:**

- Seltzer
- 100 percent fruit juice
- Water
- 1 percent or skim milk

OR

- Homemade soup or *Healthy Choice* brand soup. Choose broth-based soups as opposed to cream-based soups, which are higher in fat.
- *Reduced-fat Triscuits, Wheat Thins, or Saltines* (check package for serving size)
- Fruit (see list above)
- One squeezable yogurt

OR

- One slice large cheese pizza (order "go easy on cheese")
- Pick a veggie (see list above)
- Pick a fruit (see list above)
- Add a beverage (see list above)

OR

- One cup yogurt or cottage cheese
- One fruit (see list above)
- Sliced vegetables (peppers, celery, cherry tomatoes)
- Reduced-fat *Wheat Thins*, or whole-grain bread or roll

What's for Dinner?

Making dinner for a family with varying tastes can be daunting at times. Trying to streamline the process, prepare healthy foods, and enjoy these foods with my family of five is my ultimate goal. With proper planning, and involvement of all those who you are feeding, making health meals can be easy, rewarding, and fun. Now that you have coordinated some menu ideas and made your grocery list, consider the following:

- Look at your week ahead. Plan which days you have time for a more complicated recipe or one that requires longer cooking times; pick the best day to prepare that meal.
- On days when you get home near, at, or past dinner time, plan to make a Crock-Pot recipe that morning so dinner will be done when you get home.
- Involve the family in meal preparation, table setting, and cleanup, as these are vital skills they will use in their independent lives outside the family home. Group effort in meal planning also helps streamline or minimize the work the chef needs to be engaged in, making mealtime a more efficiently run event.

Instead of resorting to convenience dinners such as frozen chicken potpies, frozen pizzas, and other highly salted, preserved unnatural foods, try some of these quick-fix dinners when time is of the essence. These menus can be made in thirty minutes or less and the recipes can be found at the end of this book:

Chicken with sides
Oven-baked chicken tenders
Baked potatoes (cook quickly in the microwave or try smashed potatoes) (see recipe)
Bagged, organic, prewashed baby leaf salad greens with light vinaigrette (see recipe)

Meatloaf with sides
Ground turkey meatloaf (to minimize cooking time, make in small loaf pans) (see recipe)
Organic frozen mixed vegetables
Sweet potato fries (see recipe)

<u>Basic stir-fry with sides</u>
Basic stir-fry (see recipe)
Green salad
Wheat or lentil pilaf

<u>Pasta night</u>
Pasta with tomato and basil (see recipe)
Salad or raw vegetables of your choice

<u>Taco salad (see recipe)</u>
Baked tortilla chips and salsa

Planes, Trains, and Automobiles

Obstacles don't have to stop you. If you run into a wall, don't turn around and give up. Figure out how to climb it, go through it, or work around it.
—Michael Jordan

When eating on the run means having to dine outside of the home, follow some simple guidelines.

If eating in the car is the only option, consider packing a "car picnic." When time is of the essence, pack fresh sandwiches, colorful fruit, and some healthy, crunchy snacks such as baby carrot sticks, sliced red peppers, celery sticks, pretzels, baked chips, or light popcorn. It truly does not take that much time to whip up a picnic lunch. In addition, the cost savings is tremendous and avoiding fast food makes the health benefit priceless.

In the busy world we live in, planned, home-cooked meals may not always be an option. When you are in a pinch, try to make healthy choices.

Fast Food and Dining Out

Fast-food restaurants are not the only ones who serve us too much food. For example:

"Cheesecake Factory" franchise restaurant items:

- Carrot cake and others: over 1,500 calories
- Cheesecake, plain: 700 calories
- "Six carb" original cheesecake: 610 calories

When dining in a sit-down restaurant, consider the following:

- Take one slice of bread or a roll, and then ask the wait staff to take away the breadbasket.
- Ask for your salad dressing on the side, if it is not a salad pre-dressed with a light vinegar-and-oil dressing.
- Since portion sizes can be very large, don't feel the least bit guilty in leaving some on your plate or asking for a doggy bag. You might also share an entrée with someone.
- Ask for water as a beverage.

Fast food has slowly made some healthy accommodations. Salad is now an option at most of the big fast-food chains. However, not all salads are created equally, so be careful to note the individual ingredients. For instance, if fried chicken, creamy dressings and cheese are the main additions to the greens, you may be consuming a great deal of fat, salt, and calories. Keep in mind, an "extra large" meal at a fast-food restaurant can, and often does, contain sixteen hundred calories or more. At five hundred calories, a kid-size meal may be just enough to fill your hungry stomach.

Some simple guidelines for fast-food restaurants include the following:

- Choose a plain burger or grilled chicken; have them hold the sauce.
- Select a side salad vs. French fries.
- Select small fries vs. large.
- When choosing salads, choose grilled chicken vs. fried.
- Choose light salad dressing or reduced-fat dressing.
- Avoid breakfast sandwiches made with biscuits or croissants. Instead, choose an English muffin or whole-wheat bread.
- Choose breakfast items with a side of Canadian bacon, which is lower in fat, instead of bacon or sausage.

Asian Fast Food

When Asian food beckons, refer to the following guidelines:

- Choose wonton or hot and sour soup.
- Try steamed vegetable dumplings vs. fried pork or meat-based dumplings.
- Choose dishes made with water chestnuts vs. nuts
- Choose steamed vs. fried rice.
- Limit or avoid fried appetizers.
- Enjoy sushi.
- Select Szechuan shredded chicken.
- Try velvet chicken.
- Try shrimp with snow peas.
- Pick garlic chicken or shrimp.
- Order chicken or shrimp chop suey.

Avoid the following high-calorie and/or high-fat items:

- Tempura
- Peking duck
- Kung Pao chicken
- Sweet and sour chicken, pork, or shrimp
- Crispy fish
- Fried dumplings
- Sizzling rice soup
- Fried banana
- Chow mein fried noodles

Sandwich Shops

Some easy tips to make sandwich shops healthier options:

- Choose lean roast beef, turkey, or ham; grilled chicken; or vegetable sandwiches.
- Ask for only one slice of cheese.
- Opt for the shop's "heart-healthy line" (e.g. D'Angelo notes these items with a heart symbol.)
- Try mustard instead of mayonnaise.
- Ask for extra vegetables for fiber and good nutrition.
- Add a dash of olive oil and vinegar instead of mayonnaise.

Avoid:

- Chicken, seafood salad, or tuna salad subs (they are often made with full-fat mayonnaise)
- Steak and cheese subs (no need to explain!)
- Meatball subs

- Eggplant parmigiana (eggplant soaks up a lot of oil when it's fried, making this choice very high in fat)
- Italian subs

Most food chains have Web sites with valuable information about the food they serve and their nutritional content. You may also ask many fast-food establishments for their printed nutritional information right in their shop. If you like to surf the Web, check out the Web sites below. Even if you don't enjoy fast food, it can be mind-boggling to discover the number of calories in some of these items!

Resource List

www.mcdonalds.com
www.burgerking.com
www.tacobell.com
www.dunkindonuts.com
www.pizzahut.com
www.cyberdiet.com
www.fastfoodfacts.com

It's Just a Beverage

Who could have guessed that the traditional morning or afternoon coffee break (with perhaps a small baked good on the side) would one day become an unwitting opportunity to gulp enormous amounts of empty calories without even being aware of it?

Here are a few examples:

Starbucks

o *Strawberries & Crème Frappuccino® Blended Crème—whip: 570 calories/15 grams fat/9 grams saturated fat.*

- All scones: 410–470 calories/13–19 grams fat/7–9 grams saturated fat

Dunkin' Donuts:

- Vanilla Chai: 230 calories/8 grams fat/6g saturated fat
- Caramel Latte: 260 calories/9 grams fat/6 grams saturated fat
- Plain bagel: 320 calories/2.5 grams fat/.5 grams saturated fat With plain cream cheese: 190 calories/17 grams fat/13 grams saturated fat

Take Action: Menu Planning

- Preplan. Make a shopping list of favorite breakfasts, lunches, and dinners.
- Bring lunch to work or school at least three times this week
- Grill extra chicken; it makes yummy sandwiches or can be put on top of a salad for protein.
- Make your own portion-sized "snack packs" of items such as pretzels, light popcorn, corn chips, or whole-grain crackers. Although enticing for their convenience, one does not need to buy individually packaged snacks; you can make your own!
- Wash nonperishable fruit like apples and grapes at once so they are ready to go.
- Try bagged, prewashed, organic lettuce mixes or baby carrots. Always rinse again.
- Purchase colorful, appealing containers to pack your child's lunch in.
- Order or make extra pizza for a quick entrée for the next day's lunch.
- Look up two new recipes in this book that you would like to try.

- Purchase ingredients and plan on which days this week you could prepare them.
- Go to the local bookstore and purchase a healthy cooking magazine such as *Cooking Light* or *Eating Well*.
- Keep a list of all the healthy foods you ate this week.

Take Action: On Lunch

- Make a healthy brown bag lunch this week for you and/or your kids.
- Involve kids in menu planning.
- Be sure to include a vegetable and fruit choice.

Take Action: At Work

When at the office and time gets away from you, please don't go hungry! Remember to bring some healthy items to have on hand when work deadlines prevent you from getting to the employee cafeteria. Some quick fix items to have on hand:

- High-fiber cereals and low-fat milk—pour and enjoy!
- Instant oatmeal, box of raisins—add water and dive in!
- Spice of Nile brand soups (black bean or split pea)—add water and sip away.
- Healthy Choice brand canned soups. Serve with some whole-grain crackers.

These items will fill your belly and keep your mind fresh for undertaking the tasks your job may demand.

Take Action: On Fast Food

- Keep choices simple (for example, a plain burger or grilled chicken).
- Rent the movie *Super Size Me,* and judge for yourself!

Take Action: On Coffee Breaks

- Check into the number of calories per serving of beverage or baked good you normally choose. Multiply that be the number of times you have a coffee break over the course of a year. Then make an informed choice.
- Stick with plain coffee or tea. Eliminate specialty drinks.
- Save a special treat for a special occasion—not just because.

Chapter 8:
Back to Basics: Eating Real Food

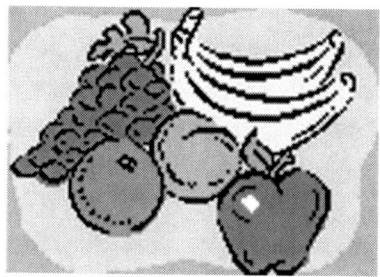

Do what you can, with what you have, where you are.
—Theodore Roosevelt

> Objectives:
> - What are the benefits of organic foods to me and my family?
> - What is Community-Supported Agriculture?
> - What should I know about bovine growth hormone? Genetically modified foods?

Of the necessities of life which the home must provide—food, clothing, and shelter—food is the most important.
—Mary Swartz Rose, *Feeding the Family*, 1940

Go Organic: You'll Be glad you Did

Every day we eat. This can be an anonymous, unplanned, utterly forgettable experience that we get through because we must, without any pleasure or thought. Or it can be a daily opportunity to show loving respect for your body and the Earth. Nothing is more important than your health, your family's health, and the world we leave to our children.

Every day we have a voice in the outcome. We can use the food that we choose to make a statement on a daily basis to emphasize these values.

Opponents of the organic food industry say that organic foods have the same level of nutrients; therefore, the food is the same no matter how it is grown. Hence, it is a waste of money to buy organically grown food items. What a sad commentary on the way our high-tech, low-touch society perceives food—not as something to be enjoyed and shared, but as a collection of nutrients to be swallowed.

Although organic and conventional foods often share the same nutrient values (to the extent that nutrients have been defined to date), organic foods do not harbor the quantity of pesticide residues. In addition, organic food items often taste better (taste a standard carrot next to an organically grown carrot for comparison), give us greater choice, and provide us with the opportunity to have a voice in a method of agriculture.

What Is Organic?

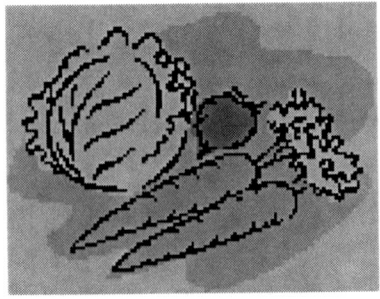

A food labeled 100 percent organic indicates that the farmer has raised the product without using synthetic pesticides, fertilizers, or antibiotics; genetically engineered seeds; irradiation; or sewage sludge. Raw products must be 100 percent organic to receive the government seal. Processed foods need to contain 95 percent organic ingredients to bear the seal of an organic product. In order for meat and poultry to be labeled organic, the animals must be fed certified organic feed that contains no growth hormone or animal by-products. The United States Department of Agriculture (USDA) defines these standards.

The Benefits

"The Best Reasons to Buy Organic"—printed on the side of every grocery bag distributed by *Whole Foods* grocery stores—says it best:

- Organic farming meets the need of the present without compromising the needs of future generations.
- Growing organically supports a biologically diverse, healthy environment.
- Organic farming practices help protect our water resources.
- Organic agriculture increases the land's productivity.
- Organic production limits toxic and long-lasting chemicals in our environment.
- Buying organic supports small, independent family farms.
- Organic farmers are less reliant on nonrenewable fossil fuels.
- Organic products meet stringent USDA standards.
- Buying organic is a direct investment in the long-term future of our planet.
- Organic farmers preserve diversity of plant species.
- Organic food tastes great!

Organic foods contain less pesticide residue, if any, as compared with conventionally grown produce. Pesticides are thought to increase risk of certain cancers, and may affect the liver and central nervous system. One can limit pesticide exposure by purchasing organic produce and by washing all produce in highly diluted liquid dish soap.

A simple rule of thumb: If you are eating the skin of the fruit or vegetable, or it has a thin skin, it is likely to contain more pesticide residues.

Conventionally grown produce most likely to contain pesticide residue:

- Strawberries
- Bell peppers
- Spinach
- Peaches
- Cantaloupe
- Celery
- Apricots
- Raisins
- Apples
- Green beans
- Grapes (particularly from Chile)
- Cucumber

Source: *Environmental Working Group; FDA and EPA data*

Produce least likely to contain residues:

- Beets
- Mushrooms
- Melons
- Squash
- Pineapple

- Oranges
- Onions
- Papaya
- Avocados
- Kiwis
- Turnips

Source: *Food Additives and Contaminants,* 220, Vol. 19, No. 5

>The best option is to eat a varied diet, wash all produce, and choose organic when possible to reduce exposure to potentially harmful chemicals.

"But organic food is so expensive. I can't afford to buy organic food to feed my family."

My friend Sue has a weekly food budget of less than eighty dollars for a family of four—soon to be five—and only purchases organic foods. I asked her how she accomplishes this, and she told me that on a typical day her family will have hot oatmeal for breakfast with dried fruit and milk. Lunch will be whole-grain pasta with cheese and raw vegetables on the side or a sandwich such as peanut butter and jelly. Dinner will usually include a piece of fish, a casserole, or homemade pizza. Her family does not eat out or get takeout. She does buy large quantities of frozen fish, vegetables, nuts, and dried fruit. She does not buy in bulk from large food warehouses like Costco.

Try spending the same amount as you do now—but shift expenses. Here are some tips for adjusting your food budget:

- Be conscious of the food you throw away.
- Prepare less, save more.
- Avoid buying in bulk if much gets thrown away or goes unused.

- Buy and prepare food in small, fresh quantities.
- Eat less meat.
- Eat less takeout.
- Prepare meals at home.
- Grow a garden.
- Use less packaging whenever possible (less plastic wrap, plastic bags, disposable containers, aluminum foil, and so on).

Eat Local

Eat locally grown and harvested foods. Supporting local farmers in your area helps sustain your community's economy and reduces the total fossil-fuel energy consumption needed to transport, refrigerate or freeze, and store the food that comes to you. Supporting local farms gives you greater choice and greater variety. Many varieties of fruits and vegetables are not available in the grocery store because they do not ship well. For example, only the hardiest of berries arrive on grocery store shelves, although they may not be the tastiest. With the absence of shipping, a local farmer can offer you different varieties than those found in the grocery store.

CSA's: Community-Supported Agriculture

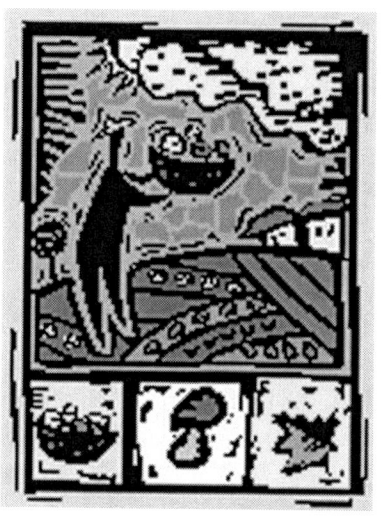

Community-Supported Agriculture, also known as CSA, is a way for the food-buying public to create a relationship with a farm and receive a weekly basket of produce. Produce can include anything that grows locally by season but can also include flowers, milk, eggs, honey, and other agricultural products. By making a financial commitment to a farm, people become members of the CSA. Most members pay for the season upfront, but some farmers will accept weekly or monthly payments. Some CSA's also require that members work a small number of hours on the farm during the growing season. A CSA season typically runs from late spring through early fall. The number of CSA's in the United States was estimated at fifty in 1990 and has since grown to over one thousand. Check the Local Harvest Web site (www.localharvest.org) to learn more about local farms, CSA's, farmer's markets, food cooperatives, and organic restaurants in your area.

What about Hormones in Milk?

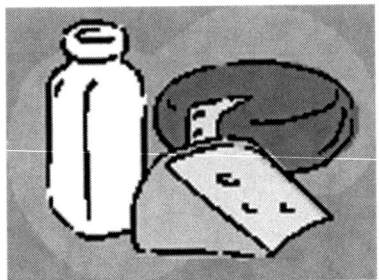

Much has been made about the use of artificial or synthetic or recombinant bovine growth hormone (abbreviated rBGH) in milk production. It is used to increase dairy cows' milk production and has no health benefit to us. It is used purely for economic reasons (to increase profit, possibly for the dairy farmer but primarily for the companies that make synthetic growth hormone).

Concerns about rBGH predominantly center on

- the safety of the use of growth hormones in our milk supply.
- the safety to the dairy cattle on which it is used.

Health concerns include whether the use of growth hormone increases the levels of insulin-like growth factor 1 (IGF-1) in our blood levels, which has been associated with breast and prostate cancers, among others.

The safety of its use in dairy cattle includes concerns about an increase in the rate of mastitis, requiring antibiotics to be given to dairy cattle and thereby increasing rates of antibiotic-resistant organisms. This ultimately impacts us all by making antibiotics less powerful against fighting infection.

The FDA (www.fda.gov) supports its conclusion that based on available scientific evidence, bovine growth hormone is completely safe—and the FDA still stands by that statement today.

At the same time, European nations take a decidedly different stand. The European Medicines Agency (EMEA) and the European Commission's *Scientific Committee on Veterinary Measures Relating to Public Health* report determined that growth hormones in meat and dairy products did not meet their standards.

In spite of the fact that most people would choose not to consume synthetic growth hormone with their milk, it is illegal for those in the dairy industry to indicate on the milk carton label that milk does not contain rBGH. (at date of printing) Today, you can find dairy brands that do not contain rBGH—it may or may not be identified on the label. However, you can often find the information disclosed on a dairy distributor's Web site. In addition, organic milk products will not contain rBGH.

What about Genetically Modified Foods?

The first time that "no GMO" entered my consciousness was shopping at an organic food market and discovering baby food labeled as non-GMO in stark black and white. However, these baby food varieties were few and far between. I explored a little further to see what I could learn. There are several terms used interchangeably to refer to crops that have been genetically modified in some way—including genetically engineered (GE) foods, genetically modified organisms (GMO), genetically modified (GM) foods, and biotech or bioengineered foods.

"Biotechnology" is a term often interchanged with "genetically modified." However biotechnology encompasses a broader range of functions. For example, biotechnology is used to make wine, cheese, beer, and yogurt. Genetically modified products take biotechnology to the next level. Since 1994, when the first genetically modified tomato designed to ripen without rotting arrived on the market, I was surprised to find that there are many unlabeled bioengineered foods currently on the market. They include the following:

- Canola oil
- Corn
- Cottonseed oil
- Papaya
- Potatoes
- Soybeans (soybean oil, soy sauce, soy products)
- Squash
- Sugar beets
- Tomatoes

Because these foods are contained in the ingredients of an enormous number of processed foods, the Grocery Manufacturers of America estimates that 70–75 percent of all processed foods available in your grocery store contain GMO's. Examples include cold cereal, crackers, breads, and even soda (it contains corn syrup made from corn, which is genetically modified).

The potential benefits of GMO's are:

- Improve pest resistance and reduce need for pesticides
- Tolerate spraying of herbicides (which also harm crops)
- Increase disease resistance
- Improve environmental tolerance to cold and drought
- Increase nutrient density of third-world countries' food staples such as rice

The potential concerns of GMO's are:

- Labeling is not required to indicate whether a food has been genetically modified or not. Safety-testing guidelines for genetically modified foods are voluntary.

- Nobody knows whether modifying foods at the molecular level will result in developing a food allergen that might be hazardous to allergy-sensitive segments of the population.

The last word comes from a 2004 report entitled *Safety of Genetically Engineered Foods*: *Approaches to Assessing Unintended Health Effects,* published by the Committee on Identifying and Assessing Unintended Effects of Genetically Engineered Foods on Human Health, National Research Council of the Institute of Medicine. Their final recommendations were as follows:

- Genetically engineered foods should undergo a safety assessment *before* being made available on the market and their evaluation should continue *after* being made commercially available.
- Genetically engineered foods should be evaluated for potential adverse effects.

Take Action: Explore Your Options for Organic and Locally Grown Produce

- Look for organic produce and other products in your local supermarket. Compare the prices between traditionally grown or manufactured produce and organic produce.
- Look for opportunities to buy locally harvested foods. For example, is there a farmer's market, local fish market, butcher, or bakery that makes organic whole-wheat breads?
- Try some new products. Get to know the local people who provide these foods. If they get to know you and what you like, it makes shopping for food that much more enjoyable. May our food suppliers become friends, as opposed to anonymous vendors.

Take Action: Compare the Costs of Organic versus Conventionally Grown Foods

With the same budget allotted, try switching to simple, home-prepared meals made with available organic or locally grown produce for a week. Try to keep within the same budget, but adjust where you spend your money.

Action: New Food Paradigm

- If you are concerned about bovine growth hormone, find out from your local grocery store what commonly available brands of milk do not contain bovine growth hormone, or purchase organic milk.
- If you are concerned about consuming genetically engineered foods, consider shopping at stores that have a policy in place against genetically engineered ingredients (for example, Trader Joe's, Whole Foods, and Wild Oats).
- Write to your local representative about your concerns related to the food supply.
- As biotechnology becomes more advanced, increase your awareness of how it may impact you and your family.

Chapter 9:

Where's the Beef? Less Is More When It Comes to Meat

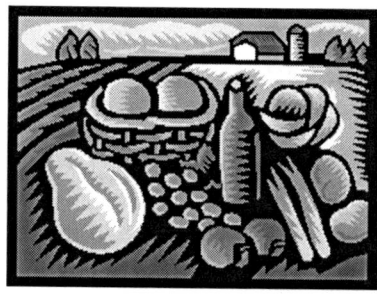

I have from an early age abjured the use of meat, and the time will come when men such as I will look upon the murder of animals as they now look upon the murder of men.

If you would keep healthy, follow this regimen: do not eat unless you feel inclined, and sup lightly: chew well, and let what you take be well cooked and simple. He who takes medicine does himself harm; do not give way to anger and avoid close air; hold yourself upright when you rise from table and do not let yourself sleep at midday. Be temperate with wine, take a little frequently, but not at other than the proper meal-times, nor on an empty stomach; neither protract not delay the [visit to] the privy. When you take exercise let it be moderate. Do not remain with the belly recumbent and the head lowered, and see that you are well covered at night. Rest your head and keep your mind cheerful; shun wantonness, and pay attention to diet.

—Quote attributed to Leonardo Da Vinci

> Objectives:
> - What are the benefits to moving from an animal-based diet to a plant-based diet?
> - What factors should I consider?
> - What about protein?

Vegetarianism

The first vegetarian I ever met was my sister. As a teen she grew tired of my grandmother's famously overcooked chicken and decided to avoid meat altogether. At first it was just an act of defiance and one that we thought surely wouldn't last. However, twenty years later, she has still not eaten a piece of meat.

From time to time her comments would annoy me. "My cholesterol has never even reached one hundred!" "Why are you feeding your kids hot dogs?" "You know I can't eat turkey if I come to your house for Thanksgiving." "Can you buy some rice or soy milk for me to have in the house when I come to visit?"

The whole concept seemed ridiculous. I was squarely in the "vegetarians are loonies" camp. This was a fringe lifestyle meant only for those on the far edges of mainstream American society. My formal education and training in nutrition implied this as well. As a cardiac dietitian, the dietary research and guidelines the experts recommended never included the suggestion that vegetarianism might be a credible option to cardiac bypass surgery. (To read more on the benefits of a vegetarian diet and its affect on reducing heart disease, read *Eat More Weigh Less* and other books by Dr. Dean Ornish). Those that did were considered extremists.

I did not understand at the time the enormous power that the dairy and meat industries wield over policymakers (see *Food Politics* by Marion Nestle). Healthcare policymakers are under enormous pressure never to suggest specifically limiting or eliminating meat or dairy products. This would be considered downright un-American!

Then my husband turned forty. He gained a lot of weight. His cholesterol level went up, as did his blood pressure. With long hours at work, he no longer had time to exercise. If this trend continued for the next decade, heart disease would be inevitable. Then we had our third child. And my husband's uncle unexpectedly died of a stroke. Suddenly vegetarianism became a very real option. It was well worth the sacrifice compared with the remote possibility that I might live a significant portion of my life without my husband, and worse, might raise our children alone.

As one who has come a long way in my response to vegetarianism, I encourage others to consider it as an option, particularly if you or a loved one is facing the potential of a family member suffering from cardiovascular disease in one of its many forms. Experiment with using less meat in your diet and see how you feel. Also, consider incorporating a meatless meal into your week of menu planning.

Assess your own risk for heart disease:

- National Heart, Lung, and Blood Institute:

   Risk Assessment Tool for Estimating Ten-Year Risk of Developing Hard CHD (Myocardial Infarction and Coronary Death) http://hin.nhlbi.nih.gov/atpiii/calculator.asp?usertype=prof
- Harvard School of Public Health: Your Disease Risk

   http://www.yourdiseaserisk.harvard.edu/

What is a vegetarian, anyway?

In general, a vegetarian is someone who avoids meat. Vegetarians come in many varieties. For example, lacto-ovo vegetarians eat milk and egg products, but not meat or fish. Flexitarians generally avoid meats, but eat them on occasion. Vegans avoid all meat products, as well as any other animal-derived product, such as dairy products, eggs, and even honey.

When giving patients recommendations for reducing cholesterol levels, it always surprised me when someone would say, "Oh, but I don't eat meat. I eat chicken, pork, and fish—just not *red* meat." In the 1990s, the pork industry began a very effective ad campaign promoting pork as the "other white meat." Somehow the meat industry differentiated animal protein into two categories: "white" and "red," when what is really meant is "beef" and "anything else."

Benefits

It is difficult to identify the specific benefits attributable to vegetarian eating, as many vegetarians also make other healthy lifestyle choices, such as not smoking, drinking alcohol in limited amounts (if at all), and eating more fruits and vegetables. They are also generally more physically active than the general population. Having said this, vegetarians as a whole appear to enjoy measurable health benefits, including a lower risk of the following:

- Heart disease
- Diabetes
- Stroke
- Some cancers
- Obesity
- High blood pressure
- Digestive disorders

If you are considering eliminating meat from your life for whatever reason, and need social support, you can find a variety of vegetarian groups out there—from singles groups to animal rights activists. Here are just a few:

American Vegan Society www.americanvegan.org

Organic Athlete www.organicathlete.org
Vegetarian Resource Group www.vrg.org
Vegan Outreach www.veganoutreach.org
Vegan Society www.vegansociety.com
VegFamily Magazine http://vegfamily.com

Protein: How Much Do I Need?

The door to success is always marked Push.
—author unknown

For most Americans, becoming a vegetarian is not a serious consideration. However, we can still reap substantial benefit from reducing our intakes of extra animal protein sources—particularly those containing saturated fat—and replacing those calories with other nutrient-dense foods like non-fat dairy products, fruits, vegetables, and whole grains.

Scientific and clinical research demonstrates that our protein requirements are met with 0.8 grams of protein per kilogram of body weight. What does this mean? It means that the average healthy woman needs fifty grams of protein to meet her daily protein needs. The average healthy man needs eighty grams of protein to meet his daily protein needs.

If you want to know your *exact* protein requirements, take your body weight in pounds and divide it by 2.2 (there are 2.2 pounds in a kilogram). Multiply this number by 0.8 to get the grams of protein your body needs. (If you have a chronic kidney disease, have a metabolic disease, are extremely obese, are a professional power lifter, or are pregnant or breastfeeding, see a registered dietitian to calculate your protein requirements.)

Your body weight, lbs./2.2 x 0.8 = Daily grams of protein needed

The average person eating a typical American diet will more than likely consume twice the ideal amount of protein daily. Since we all need to consume more fruits and vegetables for optimal health, this means that we can cut back on meat, greatly increase fruit and vegetable intake, and still be consuming the same total number of calories. We can eat more plant-based foods, eat less protein-based foods, and not gain weight! Below is a list of commonly eaten foods and the amount of protein contained in them.

Protein Content of Some Common Foods

Food Item	Grams of Protein, Average Range
8 ounces (1/2 pound) beef, ham, turkey, pork	48–64 grams
McDonald's Quarter Pounder with cheese	30 grams
1 chicken breast	50–60 grams
1 hot dog	5–10 grams
1 cup nuts	15 grams
1 fish fillet (1/2 pound)	32–48 grams
1 slice from a medium cheese pizza	10 grams
1 cup macaroni and cheese	6–12 grams
1 tablespoon peanut butter	5 grams
1 sandwich made with 2 slices bread, 4 slices deli meat, and 2 slices cheese	25–35 grams
1 cup cold cereal with 1 cup milk	10–12 grams
1 slice of cheese	6–7 grams
1 cup milk	8 grams
1 cup ice cream	4–7 grams
1 muffin, scone, or bagel	3 grams

Food Item	Grams of Protein, Average Range
1 cup fruit or piece of fresh fruit	0
1 serving meat-based casserole dish	10–20 grams
1 cup juice	0
1 cup coffee or tea	0
1 soda, seltzer, bottled beverage	0
1 cup pasta, rice, potato, squash, stuffing, French fries, or other grain	3–8 grams
1 cup legumes (refried beans, chili, soup)	15–22 grams
1 candy bar	0–4 grams
1 fortified breakfast bar	5–10 grams
1 small bag chips, pretzels, crackers	1–3 grams
1 cup fresh, frozen, or canned green vegetable	5–10 grams
1 piece cake, pie, or similar dessert	2–5 grams
1 egg, prepared in any way	5 grams

Source: Pennington and Church, 14th edition

Look at the labels of some of the foods you eat this week. What is the amount of protein per serving in those foods? If you eat out or prepare meals, try to estimate the amount of protein in those dishes. Use the previous table as a rough estimate.

Enter the estimated amount of protein you eat over the course of three days here:

Day 1		Day 2		Day 3	
Food	Protein, Grams	Food	Protein, Grams	Food	Protein, Grams
Example:					
Milk	8				
Cereal	3				
TOTAL					

- Did you meet your protein requirements?
- Did you eat more or less protein than your body needs? Try to adjust the serving size and the kinds of foods you eat to achieve the optimal amount.

Cooking Meatless at Home

Try a meatless meal this week. Some meal suggestions follow, or try some of the meatless recipes contained in this book.

Quick options:

1. Macaroni and cheese out of the box
Add salad and crusty bakery bread for a meal.

2. Frozen cheese ravioli (fresh or from the freezer section of the grocery store)
Add tomato sauce and top with parsley or grated Parmesan cheese.
Add a green salad and crusty bakery bread for a meal.

3. Vegetable cheese pizza
Buy premade pizza dough from the grocery store. Roll out the dough on a cookie sheet, or slice a piece of French bread in half the long way. Add any tomato sauce, vegetable, and grated cheese toppings. Follow the baking instructions on the bread dough package. If using French bread, put in the oven at 350° until the cheese is melted.

4. Burritos
Put a scoop of refried beans, a scoop of salsa from a jar, and grated cheese (Mexican mix is best) on a whole-wheat tortilla. Heat in the toaster oven or regular oven at 300° for twenty minutes. Take it out, plate it, and top with more grated cheese, salsa, chopped olives, sour cream, or guacamole.

Take Action

- Calculate your protein needs.
- Estimate the amount of protein you normally consume.
- Try a meatless meal or two this week.
- Assess your risk for heart disease using one of the suggested online evaluation tools.

Chapter 10:
Food Labels: How to Read One

You can't build a reputation on what you are going to do.
—Henry Ford

Objectives:
- How do I read a food label?
- How do the nutrient percentages apply to me? Members of my family?
- How can a food label of information on a food package mislead me?

Nutrition Facts

Serving Size 1 cup (228g)
Servings Per Container 2

Amount Per Serving

Calories 250   Calories from Fat 110

	% Daily Value*
Total Fat 12g	18%
Saturated Fat 3g	15%
Trans Fat 3g	
Cholesterol 30mg	10%
Sodium 470mg	20%
Potassium 700mg	20%
Total Carbohydrate 31g	10%
Dietary Fiber 0g	0%
Sugars 5g	
Protein 5g	
Vitamin A	4%
Vitamin C	2%
Calcium	20%
Iron	4%

*Percent Daily Values are based on a 2,000 calorie diet. Your Daily Values may be higher or lower depending on your calorie needs.

	Calories:	2,000	2,500
Total Fat	Less than	65g	80g
Sat Fat	Less than	20g	25g
Cholesterol	Less than	300mg	300mg
Sodium	Less than	2,400mg	2,400mg
Total Carbohydrate		300g	375g
Dietary Fiber		25g	30g

Source: Nutrition Facts Label Images for Download US Food and Drug Administration CFSAN/Office of Nutritional Products, Labeling, and Dietary Supplements

Food labeling can be daunting—even for those of us who make it our profession to interpret them. There are many times I have mistakenly bought a grocery item, only to bring it home and be horrified at the contents. For example, I once bought my kids some whoopie pies as a special treat. Since it was a one-time thing, I didn't concern myself much with the contents ... until I got home, glanced at the label, and found that each whoopie pie was intended to serve two! And since my kids each ate one by themselves, they each consumed a whopping one-thousand calorie snack with forty-six grams of fat!

Here are some basic guidelines to answer the questions: Should I buy it? Is it healthy?

- **Fat.** The total daily fat limit for most women should be thirty to fifty grams and for most men fifty to seventy grams. Take these numbers into consideration when choosing high-fat items. Recognize that a fast-food lunch can blow your entire daily fat allotment.
- **Calorie/fat goal.** For an item with one hundred calories per serving, fat should be limited to three grams. For an item with two hundred calories per serving, fat should be limited to six grams. In other words, fat calories (nine calories per gram of fat) should not make up more than 30 percent of the total number of calories.

  If a snack food contains more than 30 percent of its calories from fat, choose a lower-fat version, if it exists. For example, snack crackers such as Cheez-It brand or Cheese Nips brand crackers have a lower-fat version and a regular-fat version. One version is higher than 30 percent fat; the other is lower than 30 percent fat.
- **Saturated fat.** The intake of saturated fat increases blood cholesterol levels; therefore, you should limit your intake. Intake for most women should be twelve to sixteen grams, for most men eighteen to twenty-two grams—or not more than 10 percent of total daily fat intake. Take note: the mandatory labeling for *trans* fats on food labels has encouraged food manufacturers, in an effort to make

their food item free of trans fats, to add saturated fats in place of partially hydrogenated fats. Buyer beware!

- ***Trans* fats.** Current recommendations limit recommended intake to two grams per day or less, although they are best avoided altogether. As discussed previously, *trans* fats are a by-product of hydrogenation, a process by which liquid oils in their natural state are made harder, thereby increasing shelf life. Because foods can be divided into a small enough portion size to contain less than 0.5 grams of trans fat per serving—rounding down to zero grams of trans fat per serving—it's best to avoid products containing hydrogenated or partially hydrogenated vegetable oils in general.

- **Cholesterol.** The intake of cholesterol should be limited to three hundred milligrams per day. Compare the amount of cholesterol contained in a serving to this number.

- **Carbohydrates.** Carbohydrates should make up 45–50 percent of your total daily calories. Choose carbohydrate-rich foods that also contain fiber. Note that each teaspoon of table sugar (sucrose) equals four grams of sugar or sixteen calories per teaspoon. This is not a lot when considering adding a teaspoon of sugar to tea or coffee, but it is substantial when considering the teaspoonfuls of sugar found in most sweetened beverages. (Food purists know that most beverages contain high-fructose corn syrup as opposed to the sucrose found in table sugar. Nevertheless, it's still simple sugar and something we should limit.)

- **Sodium.** Total intake should be limited to 2,200 milligrams per day for most adults. A good rule to follow is to limit your sodium to 250–300 milligrams per food serving. There is a startling amount of sodium in prepared foods, so an awareness of the foods with large amounts is an important part of good nutrition. Because salt (sodium chloride) and sodium is something you and your family acquire a taste for, teach your kids to enjoy foods with lower sodium content.

- **Fiber.** When reading cereal box labels, set a goal of four grams or more of fiber per serving.

Check the portion size first! Remember to multiply everything included on the label by the number of serving sizes contained in the package if you plan on consuming the whole package. For example, most beverages are not sold in individual portion sizes. Most bottled beverages actually contain two or more servings per container, even though they are sold in single-serving containers.

Food Packaging: Beware of nutritional claims!

Packaging is just as important as the food label. Many times the claims made in bold letters on the box are what grab our attention and cause us to buy the product, rather than the actual food label which is regulated by the Food and Drug Administration. Food claims are loosely monitored at best. Consider the following:

- **"Natural"** or **"all natural"** food contains no synthetic or artificial ingredients, although there's no restriction on sugar. "Natural" meat or poultry is free of artificial additives and subjected to only minimal processing. "Natural" meat may still contain drug residues.
- **"Light"** food generally must have a third fewer calories or half the fat of the nonlight version—but there are still some big loopholes. Products that traditionally have been known as light, such as *light cream*, are exempt, meaning that veggies prepared in a "light cream sauce" aren't necessarily low-fat or low-calorie. Certain terms such as "lightly sweetened" aren't regulated either.
- **"Healthy"** food must meet certain criteria, including a maximum of three grams of fat, 480 milligrams of sodium, and 60 milligrams of cholesterol per serving. It also has to provide at least 10 percent of the FDA's recommended daily amount of one of the following: vitamins A or C, calcium, iron, protein, or fiber. However, the food can still contain sugar or chemicals.

- **"Fat-free"** means pretty much what it sounds like—the product contains only trivial amounts of fat (less than 0.5 grams per serving). But fat-free products can still contain a lot of calories.

   Bottom line: Check the boring ingredient list and food label when in doubt; avoid letting the marketing claims influence your buying decisions when it comes to food. Choose foods in their most natural state.

- **Made with "whole grain"** means the food may be made with a lot or a little whole grain. In fact, some cereals "made with whole grain" contain only one gram of fiber per serving—an indicator of the content of actual whole grain used.
- **Multigrain** indicates a mixture; it could be mostly refined flour.
- **100 percent whole grain** means no refined flour.
- **Whole grain** means that at least 51 percent of product is whole grain.
- **With fiber added** could mean maltodextrin, polydextrose, inulin, or cellulose.

   Bottom line: When looking for whole-grain products, look for labels that say "100 percent whole grain."

Fruit Juice, Fruit Beverages, and Fruit Popsicles

Our kids are big consumers of fruit beverages and popsicles, and I have been tricked into buying a less-than-ideal fruit juice beverage or frozen dessert in the past. For that reason, some examples are highlighted here.

Hi-C Fruit Beverages: Hi-C Blazin' Blueberry drink contains pure filtered water, sweeteners (high fructose corn syrup, sugar), apple and grape juices from concentrate, less than 0.5 percent of vitamin C (ascorbic acid), natural and artificial flavors, and citric acid (provides tartness).

"Five Alive natural citrus beverage is a delicious citrus blend of five fruit juices and other *all natural* ingredients." But "Five Alive natural citrus beverage" contains pure filtered water, orange juice from concentrate, sweeteners (high fructose corn syrup, sugar), lemon, grapefruit and tangerine juices from concentrate, natural flavors, and lime juice from concentrate.

Bottom Line: Sounds good, but it's mostly water and corn syrup, even though it claims to contain "five fruit juices" or call itself a 'fruit' beverage.

Edy's brand Whole Fruit Bars contain water, sugar, blackberry juice from concentrate, natural flavor, corn syrup, citric acid, boysenberries, pectin, vegetable stabilizers (guar gum, carob bean gum), which inhibit ice crystal growth, and ascorbic acid.

Bottom Line: It's called Whole Fruit, but it's really juice with corn syrup.

Take Action: On Food Labels

- Finding the best foods for you and your family is hard work!
- Be alert!
- Stick to the least processed foods in their purest form.

Chapter 11:
A Word about Exercise

Those who have not time for bodily exercise will sooner or later have time for illness.

—Edward Stanley, 15th Earl of Derby

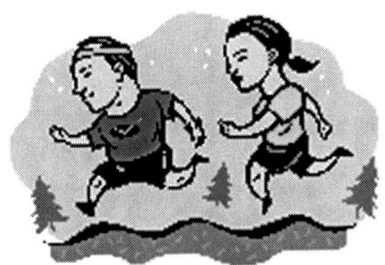

Objectives:
- What are the benefits of regular exercise?
- How can I get regular physical activity to become a part of my regular routine and my family's routine?

Moving your body is essential for good health. Exercise benefits our bodies in the following ways:

- Reduces the risk of coronary heart disease and stroke by raising the healthy cholesterol (HDL)
- Lowers blood pressure
- Reduces high cholesterol and improve levels of blood fats
- Reduces body fat

- Enhances mental well-being
- Increases bone density, hence helping prevent osteoporosis
- Reduces the risk of cancer of the colon
- Reduces the risk of noninsulin-dependent diabetes
- Helps control body weight
- Help flexibility and coordination, thus reducing the risk of falls
- Enhances ability to sleep
- Helps with socialization when exercising with others

Additionally, exercise may reduce symptoms of depression. In a study published in *the Journal of Medicine and Science in Sports and Exercise*, researchers compared the effects of thirty minutes of walking on a treadmill with thirty minutes of quiet rest in forty adults who were recently diagnosed with depression. The group that exercised reported greater feelings of vigor and well-being.

Another interesting study was undertaken by the Women's Health Initiative (WHI), a long-term national health study that focuses on strategies for preventing heart disease, breast and colorectal cancer, and fracture in postmenopausal women. The ongoing study has demonstrated that exercise is a major factor in enhancing longevity among its participants. This fifteen-year project involves over 161,000 women ages fifty to seventy-nine and is one of the most definitive, far-reaching programs of research on women's health ever undertaken in the United States.

Being active is a very important part of weight and health management. Exercise improves our body's metabolism, which is the body's way of burning energy or stored calories. Simply put, it is the speed at which your body's engine runs. We each have our own metabolism. Genetics, gender, body temperature, hormones (such as thyroid), environmental temperature, and the amount of lean body or muscle mass determine your metabolic rate or how many calories you burn.

Weight-loss diets, especially those that initiate rapid weight loss, result in muscle loss along with loss of fat. This rapid weight loss can have unfortunate long-term effects on metabolism. Muscle burns calories more efficiently than fat, so it is essential to lose weight slowly, losing primarily body fat *not* muscle weight. On any weight management program, the goal is to lose weight slowly, with diet *and* exercise as important components. Diet changes without exercise are not ideal, as you are likely to lose fat *and* muscle weight.

If one were to compare two people weighing the same amount, the one with more body fat and less muscle mass would burn calories much less efficiently, requiring the person to eat a more restricted diet (i.e., less calories). This person would need to eat far less than the person with less body fat and more muscle. Exercise will maximize muscle weight. Repeated dieting attempts without exercise lead to muscle and fat loss. When weight is regained, it is solely fat weight, resulting in a body that has more fat and less muscle than prior to the weight-loss diet. Bottom line: the dieter becomes an even less efficient calorie-burning machine.

Tips to Increase Metabolism

- **Vary your exercise routine.** Your body is a very efficient machine. When utilizing the same muscle groups each time you exercise, your body adapts and expects the same workout. This leads to less of an impact on muscle building. So, incorporate activities that utilize other muscle groups.
- **Eat six small meals vs. three large meals.** Your body uses energy to digest foods. By splitting up your eating, your metabolic rate may slightly increase.
- **Eat enough calories.** When you consume too little calories, your body responds by lowering its metabolism. Don't go on extreme low-calorie diets.

- **Weight training.** Add weights to your workout. Start with small hand weights.

Sleep well and minimize stress. Fatigue and stress may interfere with your body's ability to burn calories. Learn healthy breathing techniques, and take time to rest. If weight-loss attempts fail despite modifying your diet and exercising regularly, check with your physician to determine whether your thyroid level needs to be checked.

Make Exercise Fun!

I talk about the "pleasure component" often in my nutrition practice. It is essential to find an activity you enjoy. If walking on a treadmill and staring into space is not enjoyable to you, by all means, do not do that. Take time to find an activity that brings pleasure to your life. I enjoy jogging on the weekends with my husband. We stop for a cup of coffee on our way home. We both enjoy this ritual and have been running for years. To spice it up, we have chosen different charity runs for which to train. It may be a breast cancer fund-raiser or a leukemia and lymphoma charity run/walk. This gives the exercise deeper meaning and gives us a goal to work toward. Consider walking or running for a charity that you feel connected with. You'll be glad you did.

Kids and Exercise

> "They cut the physical education program from the schools."
>
> "My children can't play outside; they may be abducted."

Have you noticed how many children get door-to-door service to and from school? I am not talking about the bus but the parade of minivans traveling to and from school every day! The media makes us fear for our children's lives. In my generation, the neighborhood kids played outside all afternoon after school. We rode our bikes, we ran, and we played kickball, football, hide-and-seek, and cops and robbers. Children today, for the most part, have structured play, such as one hour of soccer on the weekends. With the advent of new technology, video games, computers, and television with endless cable channels, children have many stimulating activities to keep them busy but with minimal health benefits.

Sitting in front of a computer doesn't exercise your heart. Using joysticks and/or analog sticks on video game controllers does not enhance health. Yet the children of this generation spend countless hours of the day doing just that. Diet, along with this lack in activity, contributes to our country's childhood obesity problem. The majority of studies on young people and exercise indicate declining participation in physical activity.

Take Action

- Walk to school with your child.
- Find a group of kids to walk together with your child to school (safety in numbers).
- Plan an activity with the neighborhood children: basketball on Mondays, street hockey on Tuesdays, fun run on Wednesdays, scavenger hunt on Thursdays, and so on.
- Plan a family activity that involves exercise on the weekends. You might visit a local wildlife sanctuary, hike a nearby mountain or hilly terrain, or take a walk on the beach.
- Play touch football—it's actually fun! Come up with fun names for yourself and your team. Get old T-shirts and permanent markers and make team shirts.
- Consider a basketball-shooting contest.
- Sign up for a charity family fun walk.

- Walk to the local playground. Set a date each week with your children's friends.
- Join a local gym or YMCA with children's programs such as kickboxing and swimming lessons.

Are you ready to consider an exercise program? Here are some tips to get you started:

- Think of activities you enjoy now or when you were a child. Make a list. Consider swimming, basketball, walking, riding a bike, dancing, or yoga.
- Pick an activity or different activities that you could do this week.
- Put "exercise" on your calendar, just like a doctor's appointment. Keep that appointment with yourself!
- Plan on exercising for thirty minutes every day. You can break this up in increments of ten minutes or fifteen minutes or do it all at the same time.
- Get a pedometer. Keep track of the number of steps you take per day. Try to increase by one thousand every week until you reach eight to ten thousand per day.
- Get a heart rate monitor.
- Find an exercise buddy to keep you motivated, and have double the fun.
- Keep track of your exercise in a notebook.

Chapter 12:

Vitamins, Minerals, Phytochemicals, and Functional Foods: Food for Thought

We are what we repeatedly do. Excellence, then, is not an act but a habit.
—Aristotle

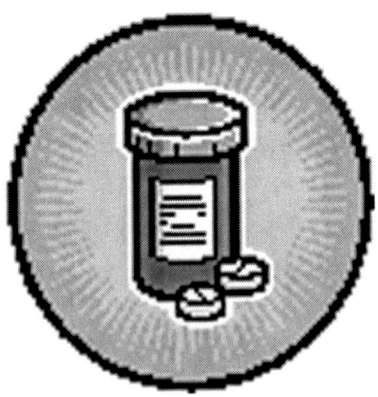

Objectives:

- Should I take a nutrition supplement?
- What factors do I need to consider if I choose a nutrition supplement?
- Are there circumstances where a less-than-adequate intake of a particular vitamin is common in the United States?

"Just before 1900, an observant physician working in a prison in East Asia discovered that beriberi (muscle wasting and/or fluid accumulation) could be cured with proper diet. The physician noted that the chickens at the prison had developed a stiffness and weakness similar to that of the prisoners who had beri-beri. The chickens were being fed the rice left on prisoners' plates. When the rice bran, which had been discarded in the kitchen, was given to the chickens, their paralysis was cured. As might be expected, the physician met resistance when he tried to feed the rice bran, the "garbage" to the prisoners, but it worked—dramatically. Later, the extracts of rice bran were used to identify the vitamin, thiamin."

—from *Nutrition Concepts and Controversies,* by Frances Sizer and Eleanor Whitney page 226.

Today in the United States, one would be hard-pressed to consume no *fortified foods,* or foods without any added nutrients. Here are just a few examples of foods with added nutrients that we take for granted today:

- Vitamin A and D added to dairy products
- Juices fortified with calcium and vitamin C
- Fluoridated water (fluoride is a mineral)
- Fortified cereals
- Thiamin, niacin, riboflavin, and iron added to grain products such as flour, rice, and pasta
- Iodized salt

We have played with the nutritional profile of most of our foods over the years, mostly to prevent debilitating or life-threatening diseases due to the lack of a particular molecular compound—for which the term *vitamin* was coined—as these essential substances were identified through scientific advances.

A Brief Introduction to Vitamins

Vitamins are molecules that function in a variety of different ways in the human body. Vitamins can be broken into two distinctive groups: water soluble (can dissolve in water) and fat soluble (can dissolve in oil).

The water-soluble vitamins are:

- Thiamin (B1)
- Riboflavin (B2)
- Niacin (B3)
- Pantothenic acid (B5)
- Biotin
- Cobalamin (B12)
- Folic acid or folate
- Ascorbic acid (vitamin C)

Water-soluble vitamins:

- dissolve in water; hence, cooking and washing reduce the amount of these vitamins.
- are easily absorbed and excreted by the body; therefore, they are less susceptible to causing harm to your body when consumed in megadoses from vitamin supplements.
- are not stored extensively in the body; therefore, you need to consume them daily in order to sustain optimal amounts.

The fat-soluble vitamins are:

- Vitamin A
- Vitamin D
- Vitamin E
- Vitamin K

Fat-soluble vitamins:

- dissolve in fat or oil.

- are stored in the body, primarily in the liver; therefore, you do not need to consume them daily as long as your overall diet averages recommended intakes.
- may be toxic in high doses; therefore, they are dangerous when consumed in megadoses via vitamin supplements.

As more research is conducted each year, our understanding of the role vitamins play and the precise amount we need for optimal health, changes.

A Brief Introduction to Minerals

The major minerals, or those predominantly found in the body, are:

- Calcium
- Chloride
- Magnesium
- Phosphorus
- Potassium
- Sodium
- Sulfur

Trace minerals, those that are found in trace amounts in the body and have recommended intake levels established, are:

- Iodine
- Iron
- Zinc
- Selenium
- Fluoride
- Chromium
- Copper

- Manganese
- Molybdenum

A Brief Introduction to Phytochemicals

Phytochemicals is a big word that means "plant chemicals." These phytochemicals often contribute the bright colors found in fruits and vegetables. A diet rich in fruits and vegetables is associated with optimal health and decreased disease risk. Because there are tens of thousands of phytochemicals and the study of them is ongoing, new benefits from individual phytochemicals will continue to make headlines. There are no recommended intake levels of phytochemicals … yet. Here is a sample of phytochemicals we know of so far:

Foods	Phytochemicals	Possible Benefits
Apples	Flavonoids	Protect against cancer, lower cholesterol
Beans, berries, black and green tea, citrus fruits, purple grapes, olives, onions, whole wheat, wine, oregano, soybeans	Flavonoids (saponins, isoflavones, flavonols, catchin, others)	Protect against cancer, lower cholesterol, bind to nitrates in the stomach
Berries	Ellagic acid	Prevent abnormal cellular changes that can lead to cancer
Broccoli, Brussels sprouts, cabbage, cauliflower, horseradish, mustard greens	Indoles, isothiocyanates and others	Protect against cancer
Carrots	Beta-carotene	Antioxidant

Foods	Phytochemicals	Possible Benefits
Citrus fruits	Flavonoids (limonene)	Antioxidant, inhibit tumor formation, decrease inflammation
Flaxseed	Isoflavones	Protect against cancer, lower cholesterol
Garlic	Allium (allyl sulfides)	Protect against certain cancers and heart disease, boost the immune system
Grains	Isoflavones	Protect against cancer, lower cholesterol
Red grapes (and wine)	Flavonoids (quercitin)	Protect against cancer and heart disease
Onions	Allium (allyl sulfides)	Protect against certain cancers and heart disease, boost the immune system
Sweet potatoes	Beta-carotene	Antioxidant
Soy (soybeans)	Isoflavones	Protect against cancer and heart disease, strengthen bones
Tea	Flavonoids (quercitin)	Protect against cancer and heart disease
Tomatoes	Flavonoids	Protect against cancer, fight infection

Source: Table c11–2: A Sampling of Phytochemicals: Classification, Possible Health Effects and Food Sources. Sizer and Whitney. Nutrition Concepts and Controversies 8th edition. 2000.

Phytochemicals in abundance are lacking in standard multivitamin supplements, but have proven to be beneficial. The best source for them continues to be plant-based foods.

Functional Foods—Trying to Enhance Mother Nature with Food Chemistry

The American Dietetic Association defines the term "functional" as a food that has some identified value leading to health benefits, including reduced risk for disease, for the person consuming it. Functional foods are foods that are marketed as having an added benefit due to a nutrient additive. It is a billion-dollar industry and one that turns food, pure and simple, into "nutraceuticals." As more functional foods enter the market, we will see more health claims on food packaging as food manufacturers push the limits of product branding and marketing health.

Some examples of functional foods include the following:

- Benecol margarine made with stanol esters, a newly approved ingredient for lowering cholesterol
- Soluble fibers such as psyllium and inulin added to everything from yogurt to pasta
- Herbal supplements like Gingko biloba and kava kava, in your bottled juice or iced tea
- Omega-3 fatty acids fed to chickens to fortify their eggs

Should I take a vitamin and mineral supplement with added phytochemicals?

Many studies link healthy eating habits to reduced disease risk and enhanced feelings of well-being. Food seems to help the body process nutrients like vitamins more effectively compared to supplements. Foods hold nutrients in a delicate balance. For example, the ratio of calcium and phosphorus in milk is the appropriate ratio for calcium absorption and bone mineralization. The form of vitamin A found in plant foods naturally—beta-carotene—will not accumulate in your body to dangerously toxic levels like a synthetic form of vitamin A might. Iron absorption is affected by other nutrients consumed with it. These are just a few examples of how nutrients affect each other. We are still learning about all of the components of food. It would be impossible to put all of the beneficial components in ideal doses in a manufactured pill. We have a long way to go before we truly understand the complexities of nutrition and the body.

According to the federal government's own reports monitoring the nutritional adequacy of the American diet, many of us fall short of the goals outlined in the U.S. dietary guidelines. In an ideal world, with fresh local produce available every season, it would be easy to meet your nutritional needs. It is possible to meet nutritional needs with an optimal well-balanced diet, but taking a multivitamin and mineral supplement may give us the nutrients we often miss due to busy schedules and lifestyles. Reluctantly, until we can all slow down, buy local produce, and eat healthfully every day, we acknowledge the potential benefits of a multivitamin and mineral supplement, chosen with care.

For this reason and the fact that there is minimal risk in taking a multivitamin for most healthy individuals, we suggest you consider taking a supplement if your diet falls short on nutrients. In addition, chronic medical problems or long-term medication use can affect nutrient absorption. It would be prudent to discuss the effect of any medical condition or medicine intake with a registered dietitian or your physician to assess the benefits of taking a nutrient supplement(s) in addition to maintaining a well-balanced diet.

How do I choose a nutrition supplement?

Nutrition supplements are not regulated. Purchasing a quality multivitamin and mineral supplement is often a stab in the dark. The U.S.

Pharmacopoeia, an independent organization that sets standards for drugs, has implemented standards for vitamins. Look for the USP label on products of companies that adhere to these standards. Keep in mind that although the Food and Drug Administration (FDA) requires vitamin and mineral supplements to contain nutrient information on a nutrition fact label, the FDA does not evaluate the quality of the supplement. For example, a study by the Center for Science in the Public Interest tested forty vitamin supplements, of which eleven failed because they were contaminated with lead, contained lower ingredient levels than the label stated, or were poorly absorbed. Supplements are not all created equal. Be sure to educate yourself about them to make the best personal choice. Keep in mind that we are all individuals, and consider the following:

- Men need less iron than children and women who are premenopausal.
- Children's needs vary from adults.
- Certain medical conditions warrant greater vitamin needs.
- Women of child-bearing age need adequate amounts of folate to prevent the risk of birth defects.
- Many adults and children do not consume adequate amounts of calcium.
- Kids need fluoride to prevent tooth decay. It may not be adequate in their diet.
- Adults and kids living in northern climates do not generate enough vitamin D year-round. Infants generally are provided with a vitamin D supplement as well.

Many different choices of vitamin and mineral supplements are available, and the market is growing steadily. Here is what you should look for:

- Be sure the multivitamin contains the USP seal. This ensures that the vitamin contains ingredients and amounts stated on the

label, it disintegrates properly for ideal absorption, and it is free of contaminants.
- Avoid vitamins with special claims such as "aids weight loss," "for active lifestyles," and so on. These claims are not regulated. For example, most women's formulas have additional calcium but may lack the necessary amount of vitamin D, which helps calcium absorption and utilization. Senior formulas may not contain the appropriate amount of vitamin B12 (25 mcg).
- Store vitamins in a dry, cool environment, not in a humid bathroom, to maintain shelf life. Always keep vitamins out of reach of children.
- Read the expiration dates. Vitamins lose potency over time and eventually expire.
- Check the serving size. How many tablets are needed to provide the stated nutrients? You may need to swallow up to six tablets daily to get the amount listed on the label.
- Look for 100 percent of the daily value for vitamins B1 (thiamin), B2 (riboflavin), niacin, vitamin B6, vitamin B12, vitamin C, vitamin D, vitamin E, folic acid, and beta-carotene or vitamin A (beta-carotene is converted to vitamin A but will not cause vitamin A toxicity).

A Profile of Some Individual Nutrients: Thoughts to Chew On

We have chosen a few nutrients to describe in greater detail. Their story demonstrates the complexities of trying to achieve the ideal nutrient balance.

Calcium and Osteoporosis

There is a widespread concern that Americans are not meeting the recommended intake for calcium. According to the Continuing Survey of

Food Intakes of Individuals (CSFII 1994–96), the following percentages of Americans are *not* meeting their recommended intake for calcium:

- 44% boys and 58% girls ages six to eleven
- 64% boys and 87% girls ages twelve to nineteen
- 55% men and 78% of women ages twenty and over

Calcium Intake Recommendations

Ages	Amount mg/day
Birth–6 months	210
6 months–1 year	270
1–3	500
4–8	800
9–13	1,300
14–18	1,300
19–30	1,000
31–50	1,000
51–70	1,200
70+	1,200
Pregnant and Lactating	1,000
14–18	1,300
19–50	1,000

Source: Dietary Reference Intakes for Calcium, National Academy of Sciences, 1997

Foods highest in calcium content include:

Calcium does not necessarily have to come from dairy foods. Soy and rice milks are fortified with calcium, orange juice fortified with calcium is available, and a large number of greens and legumes contain calcium, along with a number of other vitamins and phytochemicals.

Food Source	Serving Size	Range of Calcium, mg
Milk, all kinds	1 cup	280–300
Yogurt, all kinds	1 cup	300–450
Cheese, all kinds	1 slice	200–270
Calcium-fortified orange juice or soy beverage	1 cup	250–350
Tofu processed with calcium sulfate	1/2 cup	250
Legumes	1/2 cup	100
Turnip greens	1 cup	200

Source: Pennington and Church, *Food Values of Portions of Commonly Used Foods14th edition 1985.*

Even if you take a multivitamin, chances are it does not include an adequate amount of calcium. This means you may need to take an additional calcium supplement.

Fluoride for Kids

Kids need fluoride for healthy teeth. The primary source for this trace mineral is drinking water. Many of us live in areas where the public water supply is fluoridated. However, if you live in an area where the water supply does not contain added fluoride, your primary water source is well water, or your kids primarily drink bottled water that is not fluoridated, talk to your pediatrician or dentist about an added fluoride supplement. The American Academy of Pediatrics (AAP) recommends that you check with your pediatrician to find out whether any additional fluoride supplements are necessary.

Folic Acid for Women of Child-Bearing Age

Folic acid, a B vitamin sometimes called folate, helps prevent birth defects of the brain and spinal cord, known as neural tube defects, when taken very early in pregnancy. These defects occur in one out of every one thousand births, making them the second most common birth defect after Down's syndrome.

All women need folic acid in their diet because it works best for the baby early in the first month of pregnancy, at a time when the woman may not even know she's pregnant. Neural tube defects arise in the first days or weeks of pregnancy. Continued use of folic acid after the first month of pregnancy, and throughout your life, ensures the future good health of you and your family.

Some studies suggest that folic acid may also protect women and men from heart disease, cervical and colon cancer, and possibly breast cancer.

The recommended amount of folate for women of child-bearing age is four hundred micrograms (µg).

Good Sources of Folate

Food Source	Amount	Micrograms, µg
Liver	3 ounces	185
Lentils	1/2 cup	180
Chickpeas	1/2 cup	145
Asparagus, raw	1 cup	125
Spinach, raw	1 cup	125
Avocado	1/2 cup	70
Fortified breakfast cereals (check the label)	1 cup	400
Orange juice	1/2 cup	46

Food Source	Amount	Micrograms, µg
Winter squash	1/2 cup	69
Cantaloupe	1/2 cup	47
Broccoli	1/2 cup	39
Beets	1/2 cup	68

Iron for Kids and Women of Child-Bearing Age

Iron, one of the most abundant metals on Earth, is essential for normal human physiology. Iron is an essential component of proteins involved in oxygen transport. Iron helps prevent anemia by carrying oxygen in the blood. It is also essential for the regulation of cell growth and differentiation. Iron deficiency limits oxygen delivery to cells, resulting in fatigue, poor work performance, and decreased immunity. On the other hand, excess amounts of iron can result in toxicity and even death. Iron supplements, as with all supplements, should be stored safely away from children for this reason.

Iron Requirements by Age and Gender

Gender	Age	Daily Iron Requirement, Milligrams, mg
Male and female	Infants, 0–6 months	Breastfed infants tend to get enough iron from their mothers until four to six months of age, when iron-fortified cereal is usually introduced (although breastfeeding mothers should continue to take prenatal vitamins). Infants on formula should receive iron-fortified formula.
Male and female	Infants, 6–12 months	11

Gender	Age	Daily Iron Requirement, Milligrams, mg
Male and female	1–12	7–10
Female	13–18	15
Female	19–50	15
Female	51+	10

Many other compounds in food impact the absorption of iron. For example, tannins present in tea, fiber, and coffee decrease iron absorption, while vitamin C increases iron absorption.

Good Sources of Iron

Food Source	Amount	Milligrams, mg
Beef	3 ounces	2.9
Navy beans	1/2 cup	2.3
Tofu	1/2 cup	6.6
Clams	3 ounces	23.8
Fortified cereal	3/4 cup	3.7
Spinach	1/2 cup	2.4
Swiss chard	1/2 cup	2.0

Vitamin D for Adults and Kids Living in Climates That Have a Winter Season

The body makes vitamin D through exposure to the sun. Unfortunately, those who live in the northern part of the United States—areas that have winter—do not produce adequate vitamin D year-round. Studies show that vitamin D deficiency is a significant problem in New England in the elderly population, resulting in lower bone density, which in turn increases the risk of osteoporosis.

Vitamin D plays an important role in calcium absorption and bone health. It is essential to take fortified dairy products or citrus juices with vitamin D, particularly in the winter months of November to April when the amount of vitamin D manufactured by the body is minimal.

Vitamin D is measured in both micrograms (µg) and International Units (IUs). The table below uses both.

Adequate Intake of Vitamin D for Infants, Children, and Adults

Age	Children (µg/day)	Men (µg/day)	Women (µg/day)
Birth–13	5 (200 IU)		
14–18		5 (200 IU)	5 (200 IU)
19–50		5 (200 IU)	5 (200 IU)
51–70		10 (400 IU)	10 (400 IU)
71+		15 (600 IU)	15 (600 IU)

Reference: Dietary Supplement Fact Sheet: Vitamin D
http://ods.od.nih.gov/factsheets/vitamind.asp

Good Sources of Vitamin D

Food Source	Amount	Micrograms, µg
Milk	1 cup	2.5
Salmon	3 ounces	4.3
Shrimp	3 ounces	3.0

Take Action

- Review the vitamin and mineral chart; identify a vitamin or mineral that you do not consume in adequate amounts. Find a food source of that vitamin or mineral, and include it three times this week.
- Write down what you eat and drink for two days. Identify nutrients that you may need to increase in your diet. Choose to eat foods that will help optimize your vitamin/mineral intake.
- Try having a red, orange, green, purple, and white fruit or vegetable every day this week. It is easier than you think. An example: make a fruit smoothie by adding your choice of fruit to yoghurt in a blender and follow it up with a salad at lunch or dinner. You did it!
- Find the calcium amounts on a food label. Try to get the recommended amount of calcium in your diet. An example: 1 cup milk is 300 mg, 1 cup fortified orange juice is 300, and one 8-ounce yogurt is 400 mg. You did it!
- Eat an iron-rich food with a food that is high in vitamin C.

Chapter 13:
Food Connections: From Field to Table

Almanzo ate the sweet, mellow baked beans. He ate the bit of salt pork that melted like cream in his mouth. He ate the boiled potatoes with brown ham-gravy. He ate the ham. He bit deep into the velvety brown bread with sleek butter, and he ate the crisp golden crust. He demolished a tall heap of pale mashed turnips, and a hill of stewed yellow pumpkin. Then he sighed, and tucked his napkin in deeper.... And he ate plum preserves, and strawberry jam, and grape jelly, and spiced watermelon-rind pickles. He felt comfortable inside. Slowly he ate a large piece of pumpkin pie.

—from *Farmer Boy*, by Laura Ingalls Wilder

My kids and I would read passages like this while reading about life on a working farm in the 1800's and delight in our amazement of how much this little boy could eat at one sitting. The amount of physical labor required to sustain the farm and produce all of this bounty made a diet of this magnitude a necessity. Although most of us have little need today to regularly consume meals of this enormity, the amount of pleasure he experiences in finally being rewarded by the fruits of his labor are something we can still aspire to achieve. All of what he eats he has personally had a hand in growing, harvesting, and preparing. He is as close to his food as one can get—and from that, he derives much joy in devouring his accomplishments.

Make Your Health a Priority

- Pay attention to details such as meal planning, grocery lists, and where the food you eat comes from. Explore the freshest, most local food sources for your table.
- Obtain the highest quality ingredients you can achieve.
- Be mindful of what, when, where, and why you are eating.
- Move from simply consuming to dining with delight.

Explore and Enhance Your Experience with Food

- Experiment with other cuisines, ethnic foods, farmer's markets, and growing your own produce.
- Attend a cooking class, try a new cookbook, or try a new recipe from a cooking show.
- Take a family or group-affiliated field trip to learn about how food is prepared; it can be a fascinating experience. Some examples include ice-cream manufacturing plants, cheese-processing plants, dairies, watching maple syrup being made, you-pick orchards and berry farms, or visiting other farms open to the public that raise anything from chickens to buffalo.
- Resist today's marketing message that food is simply a collection of nutrients to be optimized with a "nutraceutical" cocktail and some extra diet supplements on the side.

Enjoy

- Eating is something all of us do several times a day. In fact, we still spend a large part of our lives obtaining, supplying, preparing, and consuming it. What better way to improve our health, well-being, and life experience than to embrace and make time for enjoying our relationship with food.

Reference List

www.mayoclinic.com
Find information on food and nutrition and what constitutes a healthy diet, healthy cooking, and healthy eating from the Mayo Foundation for Medical Education and Research in Rochester, Minnesota.

www.healthfinder.gov
Health information from A to Z—prevention and wellness, diseases and conditions, and alternative medicine from the National Health Information Center of the U.S. Department of Health and Human Services.

www.hsph.harvard.edu/nutritionsource
The aim of the Harvard School of Public Health Nutrition Source is to provide timely information on diet and nutrition for clinicians, allied health professionals, and the public.

www.eatright.org
The American Dietetic Association's online resource for timely and objective food and nutrition information for consumers and health professionals.

www.cspinet.org
The Center for Science in the Public Interest is a consumer advocacy organization whose twin missions are to conduct innovative research and advocacy programs in health and nutrition, and to provide consumers with current, useful information about their health and well-being. They also publish the popular *Nutrition Action Newsletter*.

www.fruitsandveggiesmorematters.org
The Produce for Better Health Foundation's Web site is designed to promote greater fruit and vegetable consumption.

www.mypyramid.gov
The U.S. Department of Agriculture's MyPyramid Plan can help you choose the foods and amounts that are right for you. By entering your age, sex, and activity level, the site will give you a quick estimate of what and how much you need to eat.

www.blonz.com
The Blonz Guide. A diverse and large collection of Web sites on nutrition-related topics evaluated for reliable, scientifically sound content.

www.foodsfacts.info
Fast Food Facts is a regularly updated Web site providing nutritional information about the food served at many popular fast-food restaurants. It is *not* affiliated with any restaurant or diet program (or any other company for that matter).

Recipes

www.epicurious.com
Described as the world's largest recipe collection. Although recipes require scrutiny for nutrition content, the site will be sure to increase the variety of recipes at your disposal. Nutrient content of the recipes is not available.

http://vegweb.com/recipes/
A vegetarian recipe collection and vegetarian product promotion site.

Exercise

www.shapeup.org
The mission of Shape Up America! is to provide evidence-based information and guidance on weight management to the public, health care professionals, educators, policymakers, and the media.

www.presidentschallenge.com
The President's Challenge is a program that encourages all Americans to make being active part of their everyday lives. The President's Challenge can help motivate people of all ages and fitness levels to improve.

Vegetarianism

www.vrg.org
The Vegetarian Resource Group (VRG) is a non-profit organization dedicated to educating the public on vegetarianism and the interrelated issues of health, nutrition, ecology, ethics, and world hunger. In addition to publishing the *Vegetarian Journal,* VRG produces and sells cookbooks, other books, pamphlets, and article reprints.

www.ivu.org
The International Vegetarian Union provides a multinational resource for all things vegetarian.

For Kids

www.kidnetic.com
A Web site for kids that gives facts about physical activity, healthy eating, and self-esteem in a kid-friendly way with partnerships to many professional organizations.

www.mypyramid.gov/kids/kids_game.html
The MyPyramid Blast Off Game is an interactive computer game where kids can reach Planet Power by fueling their rocket with food and physical

activity. "Fuel" tanks for each food group help students keep track of how their choices fit into MyPyramid.

School Lunch

Center for Ecoliteracy. "Rethinking School Lunch." www.ecoliteracy.org/rethinking/rsl.html

Physicians Committee for Responsible Medicine. "The Healthy School Lunch Campaign" www.healthyschoollunches.org

Other

www.quackwatch.com
This is a nonprofit corporation whose purpose is to combat health-related frauds, myths, fads, and fallacies. Its primary focus is on quackery-related information that is difficult or impossible to get elsewhere. The site is not updated frequently.

Recommended Cookbooks

The American Heart Association Cookbook series. New York: Clarkson Potter Publishers:.

> American Heart Association Quick & Easy Cookbook: More Than 200 Healthful Recipes You Can Make in Minutes (American Heart Association), 2001.
>
> American Heart Association. American Heart Association Meals in Minutes Cookbook: Over 200 All-New Quick and Easy Low-Fat Recipes, 2002.
>
> The New American Heart Association Cookbook, 7th Edition, 2007.

Katzen, Mollie. Salad People And More Real Recipes: A New Cookbook for Preschoolers & Up. Berkley, CA: Ten Speed Press. 2005.

Katzen, Mollie. Moosewood Collective. *Sundays at Moosewood Restaurant.* New York: Simon & Schuster, 1990.

Katzen, Mollie and Willet, Walt MD. *Drink, and Weigh Less: A Flexible and Delicious Way to Shrink Your Waist Without Going Hungry.* New York: Hyperion, 2000.

Katzen, Mollie *The New Enchanted Broccoli Forest (Mollie Katzen's Classic Cooking)* Berkley, CA Ten Speed Press, 2000.

Katzen, Mollie. *The New Moosewood Cookbook.* Berkley, CA: Ten Speed Press, 2000.

Katzen, Mollie,*Pretend Soup and Other Real Recipies: A Cookbook for Preschoolers & Up.* Berkley, CA: Ten Speed Press, 1994.

Madison Deborah. *Vegetarian Suppers from Deborah Madison's* Kitchen. New York: Broadway Books, 2007.

Madison, Deborah. *Local Flavors: Cooking and Eating from America's Farmers' Markets.* New York: Broadway Books, 2002.

Madison, Deborah. *Vegetarian Cooking for Everyone.* New York: Broadway Books, 2007

Ornish, Dean, M.D. *Eat More, Weigh Less.* New York: Harper Collins, 1991.

Rombauer, Irma S. Becker, and Becker. *The All New All Purpose Joy of Cooking.* New York: Scribner, 1997.

Waters, Alice. *Chez Panisse Fruit.* New York: Harper Collins, 2002.

Waters, Alice. *Chez Panisse Vegetables.* New York: William Morrow Cookbooks. 1996. Alice Waters cookbooks.

Waters, Alice. et al. *Fresh from the Farmers' Market: Year-Round Recipes for the Pick of the Crop.* San Francisco, CA: Chronicle Books, 1997.

Waters, Alice. et al. *Chez Panisse Pasta, Pizza and Calzone.* New York: Harper Collins, 1996.

Books about Food For Kids

Burns, Marilyn. *Spaghetti and Meatballs for All. New York: Scholastic Press, 1997.*

Ehlert, Lois. *Eating the Alphabet.* New York: Harcourt Booksrace, 1996.

Falwell, Cathryn. *Feast for Ten.* New York: Clarion Books, *1996.*

French, Vivian. and Bartlett, Alison. *Oliver's Vegetables.* New York: Orchard Books, Hodder Children's Books, 1995.

Freymann, Saxton and Joost Elffers. *Food for Thought.* New York: Arthur A. Levine Books 2005.

Giganti, Paul and Crews, Donald. *Each Orange Had Eight Slices New York: HarperTrophy.1999.*

Hutchins, Pat. *The Doorbell Rang.* New York: *Live Oak Media, 2001.*

Satter, Ellyn *How to Get Your Kids to Eat, but Not Too Much.* Boulder, CO: Bull Publishing, 1987.

Books on Nutrition For Kids and Their Parents

Evers, Connie Liakos. *How to Teach Nutrition to Kids.* Portland, OR: 24 Carrot Press, 20063.

Magee, Elaine. *Someone's in the Kitchen with Mommy.* Chicago: Contemporary Books, 1998.

National Heart, Lung, and Blood Association. *We Can! A Parent Handbook.*

Shield, Jodie. *The American Dietetic Association Guide to Healthy Eating for Kids.* New York: JS Wiley, 2002.

VanCleave, Janice. *Food and Nutrition for Every Kid.* New York: John Wiley and Sons, Inc, 1999.

Weinstein, Miriam. *The Surprising Power of Family Meals: How Eating Together Makes Us Smarter, Stronger, Healthier and Happier* New Tork: Steerforth Publishing, 2006.

Recipes

Spinach Pie

This is a great recipe for your family or company!
Serves 4

Ingredients:

1	10-ounce box frozen spinach
1 cup	Onions, chopped
2	Eggs
2 tablespoons	Parmesan cheese, grated from a wedge of cheese
1/4 cup	Feta cheese, crumbled
1 tablespoon	Breadcrumbs
	Few sheets phyllo dough
	Kosher salt
	Fresh ground pepper
	Olive oil
	Nutmeg, if desired
	A few tablespoons melted, salted butter, if desired
	A few tablespoons pine nuts or crushed walnuts, if desired

Directions:

- Preheat oven to 375°.

- Thaw frozen spinach and squeeze out as much water as possible.
- Sauté onions in olive oil until slightly browned (about ten minutes). Let cool.
- Put in mixing bowl with salt, pepper, spinach, eggs, breadcrumbs, cheeses, nuts, and nutmeg.
- Put in small casserole dish or nonstick loaf pan.
- Thaw a few sheets of phyllo dough (found in a box in the freezer section of the grocery store). I use the microwave defrost option to thaw it and save the rest of the phyllo dough in the package in the freezer.
- Layer a few sheets on top of the spinach mixture, brushing in between each layer with olive oil or butter and with some salt and pepper sprinkled in it. Five layers are enough to make a crust.
- Bake for one hour. Can be saved in the refrigerator and baked later.

Banana Bread

This version of banana bread incorporates extra fiber for better health.
Serves 12, 1 loaf

Ingredients:

1 cup	Sugar
1/2 cup	Canola oil
2	Eggs
1 teaspoon	Baking powder
1 teaspoon	Baking soda
3–5	Ripe bananas squashed with a fork
2 cups	White whole-wheat flour
2 tablespoons	Wheat germ, optional
1/2 cup	Chopped walnuts, optional

Directions:

- Preheat oven to 350 degrees.
- Lightly oil loaf pan
- Using an electric beater, blend oil, sugar, eggs, baking soda, and baking powder.
- Slowly add flour and bananas together. The banana will separate out of the batter if you mix the batter too much, so stop when the ingredients are just combined.
- Put batter in one large loaf pan or two small loaf pans.
- Put in a 375° oven for one hour (less if using smaller loaf pans).

Easy Homemade Applesauce

If you have small kids, you probably are familiar with finding apples with only one bite taken out of them and then put back. We leave a fruit bowl of apples out during the winter and fall, resulting in many half-eaten apples. Now here's a solution: put them in a bag in the fridge, and make applesauce!
Serves 4–6

Ingredients:

6+ Apples, any variety
Sugar, cinnamon as desired

Directions:

- Cut and core apples into small pieces. You don't even have to peel them! Apples with a red skin will tint the applesauce a beautiful pink.
- Put in saucepan with a small amount of water in the bottom.
- Boil until soft and chunky. Add sugar and cinnamon as desired.

Winter Roast Chicken Dinner

Winter vegetables with this chicken make it a uniquely winter dish. Serves 8–10

Ingredients:

1	4–6 pound free range chicken
1	Lemon
4	Garlic cloves
2 cups	Brussels sprouts
2 cups	Small onions
2 cups	Baby carrots
	Kosher salt, fresh ground pepper, fresh thyme, or dried thyme

For the gravy, a few tablespoons flour and organic chicken broth.

Directions:

- Preheat oven to 425 degrees.
- Prepare chicken: pull out giblets, cut off any extra fat or skin. Rinse and pat dry.
- Stuff chicken cavity with two lemon halves, garlic cloves, and fresh thyme sprigs or 2 teaspoons dried thyme.
- Sprinkle all over with salt and pepper.
- Put in large baking dish with all of the vegetables. To prepare Brussels sprouts, cut off base and peel off outer leaves. To prepare onions, peel and cut in half.
- Put in oven at 425° for 1 1/2 hours. Check doneness by cutting into chicken to see if juices are clear.
- When chicken is done, put it and the vegetables on a large serving platter.

- Take roasting pan and put on stove. Add a few tablespoons of flour mixed in the cup of broth. Mix scrapings from the roasting pan and broth together over low heat until boiling and thickened. Serve as gravy with chicken and vegetables.

Carmelized Winter Squash

This is a nice sweet rendition of winter squash with an added crunch from the added pumpkin seeds!
4 servings

Ingredients:

1	Winter squash (hubbard, butternut, acorn, delicate)
1/2 cup	Raw pumpkin seeds, unsalted
1/2 cup	Dark brown sugar
	Kosher salt
	Fresh ground black pepper, as desired
	3 teaspoons Olive oil

Directions:

- Preheat oven to 400°.
- Peel and cut up a winter squash into pieces that are slightly larger than mixed vegetables. Or buy squash that is already peeled and cut, and dice into small pieces.
- Place on baking sheet with a few tablespoons of olive oil.
- Sprinkle brown sugar and pumpkin seeds on top.
- Bake for 45 minutes to one hour.

Basic Granola

This makes a great breakfast cereal or topping for your favorite yogurt.
Serves 16–20

Ingredients:

6 cups	Rolled oats—plain, old-fashioned oatmeal
1 cup	Chopped nuts—any kind, preferably unroasted and unsalted
1 cup	Wheat germ
1 tablespoon	Cinnamon
1/2 cup	Canola oil
3/4 cup	Honey or maple syrup

Optional:

1 cup	Dried fruit, minced if large pieces—raisins, dried blueberries, cherries, cranberries, apricots
1 teaspoon	Grated nutmeg
1 teaspoon	Grated ginger

Other ingredients as desired: Shredded coconut, flaxseed, banana chips, carob chips, chocolate chips, white chocolate chips, butterscotch chips, and so on.

Directions:

- Preheat oven to 300 degrees
- Mix first six ingredients and spread on a baking sheet.
- Heat in 300° oven for about thirty minutes until lightly browned all over. You may need to toss occasionally while heating in the oven to get the browning even.
- Add other ingredients to suit.
- Store in a sealed jar or zip lock bag.

Pea Soup

This soup makes a filling meal when served with whole grain rolls and a salad.
Serves 6

Ingredients:

1	Onion, chopped
1	Clove garlic
2 tablespoons	Olive oil
1/2 teaspoon	Dried oregano
1/2 tablespoon	Kosher salt
1 T	Fresh ground black pepper
3–4	Carrots, diced
3	Small red potatoes, diced with skin on
1-pound bag	Dried peas
8 cups	Organic vegetable broth or water
	Croutons, optional

Directions:

- In a stockpot, sauté chopped onions and garlic in oil with salt, pepper, and oregano for ten minutes.
- Add carrots, potatoes, dried peas, and liquid.
- Bring to a boil and then simmer for 1 1/2 hours.
- Optional: Serve with croutons on top.

Turkey Meatloaf

Even if you don't like ground turkey, try this recipe you may just like it!
Serves 8

Ingredients:

1	Onion, peeled and sliced
3 tablespoons	Olive oil
3 tablespoons	Worcestershire sauce
2 pounds	Ground turkey, lean
3/4 cup	Dried breadcrumbs, plain
2	Eggs
	Kosher salt, fresh ground pepper, dried thyme (1 teaspoon), ketchup (3 tablespoons)

Directions:

- Preheat oven to 350 degrees.
- Cook onions in a pan until soft. Let cool.
- Mix all of the rest of the ingredients together, including onions.
- Form a loaf on a baking sheet. This recipe does not work as well in a loaf pan.
- I swirl a pattern on the top of the loaf with a squirt bottle of ketchup.
- Bake in a 350° oven for one hour.

Roasted Vegetables

These vegetables can be used in a variety of ways, when cold serve in a pita, wrap or sandwich. When hot, they are fabulous on top of pasta, pizza or in your favorite lasagna recipe.
Serves 6

Ingredients:

1	Eggplant, sliced
2	Onions, sliced
3	Peppers—different colors are ideal
2	Tomatoes, sliced
1	box sliced mushrooms
1	garlic clove, if desired
	Dash Kosher salt
	Fresh ground pepper
	Olive oil

Directions:

- Preheat oven to 425°.
- Spread a few tablespoons of olive oil on each baking sheet.
- Spread vegetables on baking sheets.
- Sprinkle with salt and pepper.
- Bake for approximately one hour.

Easy Blueberry Snack Cake

Serves 9

This recipe is just as easy as using a mix. Try it!

Ingredients:

3/4 cup	Sugar (you can use less sugar if you choose)
1/2 cup	Canola oil
1	Egg
1/2 cup	Milk
2 cups	White whole-wheat flour
2 teaspoons	Baking powder
2 cups	Blueberries—fresh or frozen
Optional:	Demerara sugar—a crunchy, golden brown sugar that makes a great topping

Directions:

- Using an electric mixer, mix oil, sugar, egg, and baking powder together.
- Gradually add flour and milk together, mixing on slow speed.
- Fold in blueberries.
- Pout batter into a 9 x 9 pan
- Bake at 375° for thirty to forty minutes.

White Bean Cassoulet

Meat-free and dairy-free options described below are equally as good! This recipe tastes great with turkey sausage as well for those that need a little meat.
Serves 4–6 meal size portions

Ingredients:

1 tablespoon	Olive oil
4	Shallots, sliced
2	Cloves garlic, minced or pressed with a garlic press
1	Turnip, peeled and chopped
2–3	Parsnips, peeled and chopped
3	Carrots, peeled and chopped
3	15-ounce cans white beans, any kind except garbanzo or chickpeas (for example, small white or northern), drained and rinsed
1	14.5-ounce can crushed tomatoes, drained
2 cups	Organic vegetable broth
2	Bay leaves
1 teaspoon	Dried thyme
	Kosher salt
	Fresh ground pepper
Optional:	4–6 Turkey sausage precooked and sliced
1 Tablespoon	Extra-virgin olive oil
Optional:	Parsley or breadcrumbs for garnish

Directions:

- In a Crock-Pot, add oil, shallots and garlic on high heat. Cover and let cook until softened. The length of time will vary depending on the Crock-Pot.

- Add the rest of the ingredients, and cook until vegetables are tender, about six to eight hours.
- Remove bay leaves before serving.

To serve meat free and dairy free, serve in a bowl with breadcrumbs and fresh parsley on top. Drizzle with extra-virgin olive oil.

To serve meat free, sprinkle Parmesan cheese on top in addition to the above.

To serve with meat, add precooked, sliced turkey sausage to the Crock-Pot, along with the vegetable ingredients.

Wilted Greens in Five Minutes or Less

Serves 2–4

Green leafy vegetables are a great source of calcium. Try this quick fix recipe and make your bones happy!

Ingredients:

1	Prewashed bag or bunch of fresh greens, such as spinach, kale, or Swiss chard
2 tablespoons	Olive oil
	Kosher salt
	Fresh ground black pepper

Directions:

- Add oil to the pan, and preheat stovetop to a medium heat. Add salt and pepper.
- Take out any blemished leaves and cut off stems. Cut bunch into slightly smaller pieces if desired.
- Put all of the greens in the pan—even if they are falling out of the pan. They will cook down quickly.
- Let greens wilt as you push them around the pan until cooked completely.

Homemade Baked French Fries

Try using sweet potatoes, as they are much more nutritious than regular white potatoes.
Serves 4

Ingredients:

4	Potatoes cut into wedges of desired size, peeled
2–3 Tablespoons	Canola or sunflower oil
	Optional: seasonings to try sprinkling on before baking include cumin for sweet potatoes, kosher salt and fresh ground pepper, garlic salt, Cajun seasoning, grated Parmesan cheese, or curry powder.

Directions:

- Cover bottom of a cookie sheet in oil.
- Heat just oil in a 450° oven for five minutes.
- Take out the sheet of hot oil and add the potato wedges. Potatoes will sizzle when they hit the hot oil. Be careful. Sprinkle with desired seasoning.
- Put back in oven and watch closely. Take out when browned. The amount of time they will take to bake depends on the size of the wedges cut and the kind of potato used.

Cranberry Bread

Serves 12, 1 loaf
Perfect winter quick bread packed with nutrients! It does not require a mixer.

Ingredients:

2 cups	White whole-wheat flour
1 cup	Sugar
1 1/2 teaspoons	Baking powder
1/2 teaspoon	Baking soda
1/4 cup	Canola oil
3/4 cup	Orange juice
1	Egg, mixed with a fork
1/2 cup	Chopped walnuts
2 cups	Coarsely ground fresh cranberries
2 teaspoons	Orange zest, optional

Directions:

- Preheat oven to 350 degrees
- Prepare loaf pan with small amount of oil.
- Using a knife or a food processor, coarsely chop cranberries and set aside.
- Put all dry ingredients in a mixing bowl, and blend together.
- In the center of the bowl, add oil, egg, and juice.
- Mix wet and dry ingredients together just until blended.
- Add cranberries, nuts, and orange zest.
- Put batter in loaf pan.
- Bake at 350° for one hour.

Barley Pilaf

This is a healthy alternative to the boxed varieties.
Serves 4

1 cup water
1/2 cup barley
½ cup grated carrots
¼ cup raisins
½ cup red onion, minced
2 Tablespoons olive oil
2 Tablespoons white wine vinegar

Boil water, add barley, and then simmer for eight minutes.

When barley is done, put in bowl. Mix with carrot, raisins, and red onion. Drizzle with 2 Tablespoons white wine vinegar and 2 tablespoons olive oil. Mix and enjoy.

Mushroom and Barley Soup

Barley is a great source of soluble fiber, the fiber that helps lower our blood cholesterol. Enjoy this heart healthy soup with whole grain rolls and a garden salad.
Serves 4–6

Ingredients:

1 cup barley
1 1/2 tablespoons olive oil
2 medium yellow onions, diced
1/2 teaspoon salt
1/4 teaspoon pepper
1 large carrot, sliced
20 ounces mushrooms, sliced
5 cups low-fat chicken broth
2 bay leaves
6 sprigs fresh thyme, chopped

Directions:

- In medium pan, bring the barley and four cups water to boil. Cover and reduce heat to medium. Simmer until tender, about thirty to forty minutes.
- In another large pot, heat oil over medium-high heat. Add onions and salt and pepper. Cover until onions soften. Add carrot and celery, and cook covered for six more minutes. Add mushrooms and increase heat until they have released their juices, about four minutes. Add broth, bay leaves, and thyme. Simmer ten minutes. Add barley and cook for five minutes. Discard bay leaves before serving.

Quick-Fix Turkey Meat Loaf

This is an alternative to our other turkey meatloaf recipe. This recipe has a nice vegetable flavor and is very easy to make. To shorten the cook time on this recipe, use mini loaf pans and cook for 30 minutes or until the turkey is no longer pink.
Serves 4

Ingredients:

1 packet Knorr's vegetable soup mix
1 pound ground turkey breast
2 egg whites
1/2 cup breadcrumbs
1 small yellow onion, diced
1 garlic clove, minced

Directions:

Preheat oven to 350°.
Mix all ingredients. Place in lightly oiled loaf pan. Bake for one hour or until cooked through.

Chicken and Grape Salad

Serves 12–14
This recipe can be easily cut in half.

Ingredients:

3 1/2 pounds poached or grilled chicken breast
5 ribs celery, chopped
1 1/2 cups seedless grapes (red or green) cut in half
1 1/2 teaspoons thyme
1 1/2 teaspoons garlic salt
2 cups light mayonnaise
Juice from 2 lemons
This may be served with lettuce or whole-wheat pita and wraps so be sure to have on hand what you would like to serve it with.

Directions:

Cut chicken in chunks. Add the rest of the ingredients except grapes. Mix well. Fold in grapes. Enjoy over lettuce greens or in a whole-grain pita or wrap.

Apple and Pear Salad with Cider Dressing

This is a great salad to enjoy anytime, but especially in the fall when the apples and pears are the freshest.
Serves 4

Ingredients:

Cider dressing:
2 tablespoons olive oil
1 tablespoon apple cider
1 tablespoon apple cider vinegar
1 tablespoon honey

Salad:

1/3 cup pecan halves
1 bunch romaine lettuce, washed and dried
2 red apples, halved, cored, and thinly sliced
2 pears, halved, cored, and thinly sliced
3 ounces blue cheese, crumbled

Directions:

Preheat oven to 350°. Prepare cider dressing and shake well. Toast pecans on baking sheet in oven for seven minutes. Arrange lettuce on chilled platter, and then arrange apple and pear slices on top. Sprinkle with blue cheese and nuts. Shake dressing, and drizzle over salad.

Spinach, Brie, and Walnut Salad

This is a great summer lunch meal. Enjoy this salad with crusty whole grain rolls.
Serves 6–8

Ingredients:

1/4 cup olive oil
1 1/2 tablespoons white wine vinegar
8 cups baby spinach leaves, washed
1/2 cup red onion, thinly sliced
6 ounces Brie cheese, diced at room temperature
1/2 cup toasted walnut pieces
Optional side to this salad-Brie toast
1 small loaf French bread
1 small (1/4 pound) piece of Brie cheese

Directions:

Whisk oil and vinegar to blend. Season with salt and pepper. Combine spinach, onion, and cheese. Toss dressing over salad. Sprinkle with walnuts.

Brie Toast

Preheat oven to broil.
Slice French bread
Spread with Brie.
Place on cookie sheet in oven until cheese melts-approximately 2 minutes.

Beef and Barley Soup

This is a hearty version of barley soup.
Serves 4–6

Ingredients:

1-pound extra-lean ground beef
2 cups water
2, 14 ½ oz. cans light beef broth
1, 14 ½ oz. can stewed tomatoes
1 6 ounce can V-8
1/3 cup split peas
1/3 cup barley
1/2 cup onion, chopped
3/4 cup celery, including leaves, chopped
1/2 cup carrots, sliced
1/4 teaspoon oregano
1/4 teaspoon pepper
1 bay leaf
Tabasco, to taste

Directions:

Brown meat in large stockpot, and drain if necessary. Add all ingredients except carrots and celery. Bring to a boil. Reduce heat and simmer thirty minutes. Add vegetables, cover, and simmer one hour.

Butternut Squash, Rosemary, Spinach, and Parmesan Risotto

This makes a great healthy meal or side dish.
Serves 8

Ingredients:

7 cups low-salt, low-fat chicken broth
3 tablespoons olive oil
1 1/4 cups finely chopped onion
1 (2-pound) butternut squash, cubed in one-inch chunks
2 teaspoons fresh rosemary, chopped—divided
2 cups Arborio rice
1/2 cup dry white wine
4 cups baby spinach, washed
1/2 cup 1 percent milk
1/4 cup freshly grated Parmesan cheese

Directions:

Bring broth to boil. In separate large sauté pan, sauté onion and oil about five minutes. Add squash and 1 1/2 teaspoons rosemary, and sauté about four minutes. Add rice, and sauté about two minutes, while stirring. Add wine and simmer for one minute. Add 1 cup of hot broth to the rice at a time. Allow the broth to be absorbed before adding more broth. Continue adding broth 1 cup at a time until the broth is used up. Be patient, this takes a bit of time, but the creamy end result is worth your hard work! Stir frequently and cook for about twenty minutes. Stir in spinach, until leaves are wilted but nicely green. Add milk and Parmesan cheese. Season with pepper and sprinkle with remaining chopped fresh rosemary. Enjoy!

White Chicken Chili

This is a great recipe for a crowd, just double the recipe.
Serves 6–8

Ingredients

1 pound boneless, skinless chicken breast cut in bite-size pieces
1-tablespoon olive oil, if cooking on stove.
3, 14-ounce cans light chicken broth
1, 14 ounce can black-eyed peas, drained and rinsed
1, 14 ounce can cannellini beans, drained and rinsed
1 tablespoon chili powder
2 teaspoons cumin
1 small yellow onion, diced
1 garlic clove, minced
dash of white pepper and salt
½ cup chopped fresh cilantro, optional
2 cups reduced fat grated cheddar cheese, optional
Baked tortilla chips, optional

Directions:

Easy Crock-Pot method:

Put all ingredients in Crock-Pot, and cook for four to six hours until chicken is cooked through. Pour into soup bowl, and cover with small amount (1/4 cup grated cheese). Enjoy with baked tortilla chips. If desired, top each bowl of chili with chopped cilantro.

Or

Stovetop method:

Sauté chicken in olive oil until cooked through. Add the rest of the ingredients except cilantro and cheese. Simmer for at least twenty to thirty minutes, although it can simmer for an hour on low heat. Serve in soup bowls, cover with 1/6 cup grated cheese, and cilantro if desired. Enjoy with baked tortilla chips for dipping.

Roasted New Potatoes

A tasty side dish for any meal.
Serves 5

Ingredients:

10 small red potatoes, unpeeled but poke with a knife so they don't explode in your oven!
2 tablespoons olive oil
1 teaspoon salt
1/4 teaspoon pepper
1 red onion, diced very small
3/4 cup chicken stock

Directions:

Preheat oven to 425°. Scrub potatoes. Combine oil, salt, and pepper. Place potatoes in roasting pan and drizzle with oil mixture. Move potatoes around to cover them in mixture. Bake for twenty minutes. Then sprinkle potatoes with onion and chicken stock. Bake until cooked through, about sixty to ninety minutes. Shake pan occasionally to move potatoes around.

Sweet Potato Fries

Serves 2

Ingredients:

1 large sweet potato, cut in steak-fry shapes
2 tablespoons olive oil
dash of salt and pepper
1/2 teaspoon paprika

Directions:

Lightly coat a cookie sheet with olive oil. Mix potatoes with olive oil and seasonings in bowl. Make sure to coat potatoes evenly with mixture. Place on even layer on cookie sheet and then in preheated 400° oven. Bake for seven minutes each side or until cooked through. They should be fork-tender.

Beef Stew

This stew is a great winter meal. To make a complete meal, serve with crusty bread and a salad.
Serves 4–6

Ingredients:

1 pound lean stew beef, cut in bite-size chunks
1, 12 ounce package baby carrots, rinsed
8 ounces frozen peas
2, 14 ½ ounce cans beef broth, low-fat and low-sodium
1 small yellow onion, diced
1, 14-ounce can diced tomatoes
4 ounces red wine—any kind will do.
1 tablespoon Worcestershire sauce
1/2-cup flour
4 red potatoes cut in chunks

Directions:

Add all ingredients to a Crock-Pot and mix. Cook on low for four to six hours. Ten minutes prior to eating, add peas.

Quick fix option-Put all ingredients except peas in a crockpot the night before. Keep covered in your refrigerator. In the morning, put crock-pot on its base, cook on high while you get ready for work-or your daily schedule. Cook on high for ½ hour, and then reduce to low heat. When you get home, add the peas about 10 minutes prior to eating.

Carrots and Parsley

This makes a terrific side dish.

Ingredients:

1 1/2 quarts water
5 cups carrots, thinly sliced
3 tablespoons fresh parsley, chopped
1 tablespoon honey
Dash salt and pepper

Directions:

Bring water to boil in large saucepan. Add carrots, and cook for twenty minutes until tender. Drain. Toss honey and parsley over carrots. Add a dash of pepper and salt.

Chicken Piccata

This is a great Italian dish. It tastes terrific served over linguini or rigatoni. Serve a salad to add balance and color to this yummy meal.
Serves 4–6

Ingredients:

4–6, thinly sliced chicken breasts
3 tablespoons olive oil, divided
1/2 cup flour for dredging
1/2 cup dry white wine
8 ounces low salt chicken broth
Juice of 1 lemon
2, 4–5 ounce jars marinated artichoke hearts
1 tablespoon butter
2 tablespoons fresh parsley
½ pound of your favorite pasta-optional

Directions:

If you would like to serve this dish over pasta, boil water in preparation of cooking the pasta. Cook according to the box directions.

While the water is getting ready to boil, start cooking the chicken. In large skillet, heat 2 Tablespoon olive oil over medium heat. Put thin chicken breast in clean, plastic bag with flour. Shake chicken with flour to coat. Do this with each breast individually. Place chicken in skillet that has been heating over medium heat. Sauté each breast, approximately five minutes each side, or until no longer pink. Remove chicken from pan. Add wine, chicken broth and lemon juice, and simmer for 2 minutes. Add marinated artichokes over low heat. Add butter and 1 Tablespoon olive oil, and stir mixture. Add back chicken. Garnish with fresh parsley if desired. Serve immediately.

Lemon and Mustard Chicken with Thyme

The lemon and thyme infuse very nice flavor into the chicken. Enjoy this entrée with brown rice and a side of your favorite vegetable.
Serves 4

Ingredients:

3 tablespoons flour
1/2 teaspoon salt
1/4 teaspoon pepper
4 skinless, boneless chicken breasts (about 1 pound)
3 tablespoons olive oil
1 medium onion, diced
1 cup chicken stock/broth
3 tablespoons fresh lemon juice
2 tablespoons of grainy or Dijon mustard.
1/2 teaspoon dried thyme (or 1 tablespoon fresh thyme)

Serving options include—barley pilaf (see recipe) and a side of broccoli.

Directions:

In a plastic bag, combine flour, salt, and pepper. Add chicken and shake to coat. Remove chicken and reserve excess flour mixture.

In skillet, warm 1 tablespoon olive oil. Add chicken and brown one side by cooking about five minutes over medium heat. Add another tablespoon of olive oil, and flip chicken to cook other side. Transfer chicken to plate. Add onion to skillet. Add last tablespoon of olive oil. Stir and cook onion until translucent. Mix reserved flour mixture with chicken stock. Add chicken stock mixture to skillet, raising temperature to medium high to boil the mixture and make it thicker. Then add lemon juice, mustard and dried thyme and continue stirring. As sauce thickens, bring temperature back down to medium-low and add the chicken. Simmer for about five minutes. Then remove from heat and enjoy with barley pilaf and a side of broccoli.

Pumpkin Bread

This is a great high fiber version of pumpkin bread. The flaxseeds are a great source of the heart healthy omega 3 fatty acids.
Serves 12, 1 loaf

Ingredients:

2 1/2 cups flour
1/8 cup flaxseed meal
1/8 cup wheat germ
1 1/2 cups sugar
2 teaspoons baking soda
1, 15 ounce can pumpkin
3/4 cup vegetable oil
3 eggs, beaten
1/2 teaspoon nutmeg
1/2 teaspoon cinnamon
1/2 teaspoon allspice
3/4 cup chopped walnuts, optional

Directions:

- Preheat oven to 350°.
- Prepare 2 loaf pans with small amount of oil or use nonstick pans.
- Sift together flour, flaxseed meal, wheat germ, sugar, and baking soda.
- Mix pumpkin, oil, eggs, and spices in a separate bowl.
- Combine with dry ingredients just until mixed; do not over stir.
- Stir in nuts.
- Pour into two bread loaf pans. Bake forty-five to fifty minutes, until a straw comes out clean.

Smashed Potatoes

A great side dish for any meal, but especially nice with a chicken dinner or turkey meatloaf.
Serves 6

Ingredients:

6 medium red potatoes, washed and cut in half
1–2 fresh garlic cloves
Dash salt and pepper (optional)
1/2 cup 1 percent milk
1 tablespoon olive oil
2 tablespoons butter blend, such as Land O' Lakes spreadable butter

Directions:

Fill large saucepan with water, and add cut potatoes and garlic. Put on stovetop over high heat until boiling. Boil for about ten minutes or until fork-tender. Drain water when potatoes are done cooking. Place saucepan back on stovetop but shut off heat. Smash potatoes and garlic with a potato masher. Add milk and olive oil and butter blend. If not warm enough, restart stove to warm them up a bit. Season with salt and pepper.

Black Bean and Corn Salad/Salsa

This recipe is tasty as a dip served with baked tortilla chips but may also be served as a side salad.
Serves 8

Ingredients:

1 (14 1/2-ounce) can of black beans, drained and rinsed
1 cup frozen corn, defrosted
1/2 red onion, diced in small pieces
1/2 red pepper, diced in small pieces
½ green pepper, diced in small pieces
1–2 tomatoes, diced
1/4 cup Italian dressing
1–2 Tablespoons fresh chopped cilantro, optional
Baked tortilla chips, optional

Directions:

Mix first 7 ingredients. Add cilantro if desired. Serve and enjoy.

Mexican Lasagna

This is a kid favorite. The beans add a nice source of protein and fiber to this great dish. Enjoy with a garden salad.
Serves 6

Ingredients:

1-package corn tortillas
1 lb. ground turkey breast
1 tablespoon olive oil
1, 15 1/2-ounce can kidney beans, drained and rinsed
1 tablespoon chili powder
2 teaspoons cumin
1 small yellow onion, diced
1 green pepper, diced (optional)
1, 8 ounce package reduced-fat, grated cheddar cheese
1 bottle taco sauce
1 (14 1/2-ounce) can diced tomatoes with green chilies

Directions:

Preheat oven to 350 degrees.
Brown turkey meat in skillet with olive oil until cooked through and crumbly. Season with chili powder and cumin. Add onion and pepper, and sauté until onion is translucent. Add drained kidney beans, tomatoes, and taco sauce. Simmer for five to ten minutes on low heat.

Slightly oil a 9 x 13 casserole dish. Put small amount of meat mixture on bottom of pan, and then layer corn tortillas on top. Next layer meat sauce and 1/2 cup of grated cheese. Repeat until meat sauce is gone. Finish with meat sauce and a final layer of cheese for the top layer. Cook at 350° degrees for twenty minutes, or until cheese is melted and the tortillas are heated through.

Pumpkin Soup

Pumpkin is a great source of fiber and Vitamin A. This soup is chockful of great nutrition and tastes even better.
Serves 8

Ingredients:

1 teaspoon olive oil
1/2 cup onion, chopped
1 teaspoon ginger
1 garlic clove, minced
1 1/2 cups apple cider
1/4 cup maple syrup
2 (14ounce) cans pumpkin
1 can light chicken broth
2 cups 1 percent milk
1 teaspoon flour
½ cup chopped parsley, for garnish
Ground pepper for garnish

Directions:

Coat pan with teaspoon olive oil. Heat large saucepan over medium heat. Add onion and garlic. Sauté until slightly brown. Add ginger. Stir in maple syrup, pumpkin, chicken broth, and cider. Bring to boil. Reduce heat and simmer for five minutes.

Add milk and flour, and stir over low heat until thoroughly mixed.

Garnish with fresh parsley and dash of pepper.

Special Herb Iced Tea

Serves 4

This is a tasty low calorie beverage when you desire something other than water.

Ingredients:

3 bags herbal tea (such as chamomile, peppermint, lemon, or rosehip)
1 bag black tea
4 cups boiling water
1 cup 100 per cent juice-cranberry/apple or grape juice
4 sprigs fresh mint-optional garnish

Directions:

Simmer tea bags in boiling water. Add juice while still hot. Refrigerate mixture. Serve cold with sprig of fresh mint.

Eggplant Parmesan (adapted from the *Moosewood Cookbook* by Mollie Katzen)

I serve this with whole-wheat spaghetti with tomato sauce and a green salad.

Ingredients:

1 eggplant, washed and thinly sliced
4–6 small summer squash or zucchini
Whole or sliced mushrooms, if desired
Dried breadcrumbs, plain or seasoned, or wheat germ
Flour, any kind
2 eggs, beaten
Shredded cheese, mozzarella and Parmesan combined or prepackaged Italian mix
Olive oil

Directions:

First dip the eggplant slices in beaten egg, then flour, and then breadcrumbs. Do the same for the squash.
Put eggplant and squash on a baking sheet with a few tablespoons of olive oil. Bake at 350° for twenty to thirty minutes until softened.
They will become slightly browned in the oil and will also be softened from baking.

Take off baking sheet and layer the eggplant and squash in a casserole dish. Intersperse mushrooms if you like. Add a layer of tomato sauce on top of each layer of vegetables, and top with a layer of cheese. Sprinkle with dried oregano. Bake at 350° for thirty minutes. Serves four.

Basic Stir-Fry

A quick and easy Asian dish.

Ingredients:

1 bag stir-fry vegetables
1 T. olive oil
1 pound boneless chicken, lean beef, lean pork, or shrimp
½ cup teriyaki sauce
¼ cup orange juice

Directions:

- Slice meat or clean shrimp.
- Put meat or shrimp in bowl-top with teriyaki sauce and orange juice-mix to be sure meat/shrimp is covered in sauce.
- Cover w/plastic wrap and marinate for at least 2 hours.
- Add 1-tablespoon olive oil in skillet. Place over medium high heat. Add meat or shrimp. Cook until shrimp is pink about 5 minutes or chicken is no longer pink about 8–10 minutes.
- Remove meat from skillet; add vegetables and 2 Tablespoons water. Stir over medium high heat until al dente. Add back meat to reheat. Serve immediately.
- Or for a great time-saver, cut meat when you purchase it, place in a freezer-safe plastic bag, add the marinade directly to the meat, and freeze. In the morning, remove the bag from the freezer and place in the refrigerator. When you get home, the meat should be nicely marinated and ready to be cooked!

Taco Salad

A tasty Mexican style salad.
Serves 4–6

Ingredients:

1 pound ground turkey breast
1 T. olive oil
1 T. chili powder
1 tsp cumin
Dash of salt and pepper
1 bunch red leaf lettuce, washed and chopped
1 tomato, diced
1 cucumber, diced
1 green onion, sliced
½ cup reduced fat grated cheddar cheese, (e.g. Sargento reduced fat grated cheddar)
Your favorite Italian dressing (oil based)
10 baked tortilla chips, broken in to large pieces.

Directions:

- Brown meat in olive oil. Add in spices and salt and pepper. Sauté until meat is crumbly and no longer pink. Break apart meat while it is cooking with a fork or spatula to keep the meat finely crumbled.
- Wash salad ingredients. Put lettuce, tomato, cucumber and green onion in large salad bowl. Toss salad ingredients to mix. Top with meat. Then sprinkle cheese over meat mixture. Top with the tortilla chips on top. Serve with dressing on the side. Add as desired.

Pasta with Tomato and Basil

Serves 6–8

Ingredients:

1 box whole-wheat blend pasta
4 ripe tomatoes, chopped
1 cup fresh basil, chopped
1/4 cup olive oil
Dash salt, pepper
1 garlic clove, minced

Directions:

Mix all ingredients except the pasta; let sit while making pasta.
Drain pasta; put uncooked sauce on hot pasta, and mix. Add shredded Parmesan, if desired.

Fruit Smoothie

This is a great beverage to enjoy after a good walk or work out session. Serves 2

Ingredients:

1 cup frozen 100% fruit (no added sugar)-any type that appeals to you
½ cup low fat plain or vanilla yogurt
½-frozen banana
Water to thin

Directions:

Place all ingredients in blender. Pulse blender on an off. Add water to thin to desired consistency. Enjoy.

Quick fix baked chicken tenders

These take minutes to prepare and minutes to cook. They are a favorite for kids and adults too!
Serves 4–5

Ingredients:

1 pound uncooked chicken tenders
Shake n Bake brand extra crispy mix

Directions:

Mix and bake according to package.
Make extra and serve for lunch the next day. Make a great topping for pasta or a salad. Kids enjoy these in their lunch boxes too!

BMI Chart for Adults

Body Mass Index (BMI) Table

BMI	19	20	21	22	23	24	25	26	27	28	29	30	31	32	33	34	35
Height										*Weight (in pounds)*							
4'10" (58")	91	96	100	105	110	115	119	124	129	134	138	143	148	153	158	162	167
4'11" (59")	94	99	104	109	114	119	124	128	133	138	143	148	153	158	163	168	173
5' (60")	97	102	107	112	118	123	128	133	138	143	148	153	158	163	168	174	179
5'1" (61")	100	106	111	116	122	127	132	137	143	148	153	158	164	169	174	180	185
5'2" (62")	104	109	115	120	126	131	136	142	147	153	158	164	169	175	180	186	191
5'3" (63")	107	113	118	124	130	135	141	146	152	158	163	169	175	180	186	191	197
5'4" (64")	110	116	122	128	134	140	145	151	157	163	169	174	180	186	192	197	204
5'5" (65")	114	120	126	132	138	144	150	156	162	168	174	180	186	192	198	204	210
5'6" (66")	118	124	130	136	142	148	155	161	167	173	179	186	192	198	204	210	216
5'7" (67")	121	127	134	140	146	153	159	166	172	178	185	191	198	204	211	217	223
5'8" (68")	125	131	138	144	151	158	164	171	177	184	190	197	203	210	216	223	230
5'9" (69")	128	135	142	149	155	162	169	176	182	189	196	203	209	216	223	230	236
5'10" (70")	132	139	146	153	160	167	174	181	188	195	202	209	216	222	229	236	243
5'11" (71")	136	143	150	157	165	172	179	186	193	200	208	215	222	229	236	243	250
6' (72")	140	147	154	162	169	177	184	191	199	206	213	221	228	235	242	250	258
6'1" (73")	144	151	159	166	174	182	189	197	204	212	219	227	235	242	250	257	265
6'2" (74")	148	155	163	171	179	186	194	202	210	218	225	233	241	249	256	264	272
6'3" (75")	152	160	168	176	184	192	200	208	216	224	232	240	248	256	264	272	279

Source: Evidence Report of Clinical Guidelines on the Identification, Evaluation, and Treatment of Overweight and Obesity in Adults, 1998. NIH/National Heart, Lung, and Blood Institute (NHLBI)

Centers for Disease Control and Prevention
United States Department of Health and Human Services

For adults, overweight and obesity ranges are determined by using weight and height to calculate a number called the "body mass index" (BMI). BMI is used because, for most people, it correlates with their amount of body fat.

An adult who has a BMI between 25 and 29.9 is considered overweight. An adult who has a BMI of 30 or higher is considered obese.

BMI Is Used Differently with Children than It Is with Adults

In children and teens, body mass index is used to assess underweight, overweight, and risk for overweight. Children's body fatness changes over the years as they grow. Also, girls and boys differ in their body fatness as they mature. This is why BMI for children, also referred to as BMI-for-age, is gender and age specific. BMI-for-age is plotted on gender-specific growth charts. These charts are used for children and teens two to twenty years of age. For the 2000 CDC Growth Charts and additional information, visit CDC's National Center for Health Statistics at http://www.cdc.gov/growthcharts/

Each of the CDC BMI-for-age gender-specific charts contains a series of curved lines indicating specific percentiles. Healthcare professionals use the following established percentile cutoff points to identify underweight and overweight in children.

Underweight	BMI-for-age < 5th percentile
Normal	BMI-for-age 5th percentile to < 85th percentile
At risk of overweight	BMI-for-age 85th percentile to < 95th percentile
Overweight	BMI-for-age > 95th percentile

Bibliography

Arnett, Alison. "Meet the New Kid: The Flexitarian." *The Boston Globe*. October 27, 2004.

Ashworth, Carolyn, MD. *Defeating the Child Obesity Epidemic*. Texas: PSG Books, 2005.

Ben, Linda. "Genetic Engineering: The Future of Foods." *FDA Consumer*, November–December 2003.

Benson, Herbert, M.D., and Eileen M. Stuart. *Wellness Book: The Comprehensive Guide to Maintaining Health and Treating Stress-Related Illness.* New York: Simon and Schuster, 1993.

Benson, Herbert, M.D. *The Relaxation Response.* New York: William Morrow and Company, 1975.

Butters, Maryjane. *Mary Jane's Ideabook Cookbook.* New York: Clarkson Potter Publishing, 2005.

Brown, Melody J. et al. Carotenoid bioavailability is higher from salads ingested with full-fat than with fat-reduced salad dressings as measured with electrochemical detection American Journal of Clinical Nutrition, Vol. 80, No. 2, 396–403, August 2004

Brownell, Kelly PhD. Food Fight: The inside story of the food industry, America's obesity crisis, and what we can do about it. McGraw Hill Publishing, 2004.

Campbell, T. Colin, et al. *The China Study: The Most Comprehensive Study of Nutrition Ever Conducted and the Startling Implications for Diet, Weight Loss and Long-Term Health.* Texas: Benbella Books, 2004.

Centers for Disease Control National Center for Health Statistics. "Prevalence of Overweight and Obesity among Adults: United States, 2003–2004." http://www.cdc.gov/nchs/products/pubs/pubd/hestats/overweight/overwght_adult_03.htm.

Centers for Disease Control and Prevention: Overweight and Obesity definitions http://www.cdc.gov/nccdphp/dnpa/obesity/defining.htm

Centers for Disease Control and Prevention:National Center for Health Statistics http://www.cdc.gov/nchs/products/pubs/pubd/hestats/hestats.htm

Center for Ecoliteracy. "Rethinking School Lunch." http://www.schoollunchinitiative.org/

The Center for Health and Healthcare in Schools, School of Public Health and Health Services, The George Washington University. http://www.healthinschools.org/

Cohen, Paula Hartman. "Trans Fats: The Story Behind the Label." *Harvard School of Public Health Review,* Spring 2006.

Department of Agriculture's Nutrient Database Web site: http://www.nal.usda.gov/fnic/cgi-bin/nut_search.pl.

Duyff, Roberta Larson. *American Dietetic Association Complete Food and Nutrition Guide.* New York: John Wiley and Sons, 2006.

Ely, Leanne. *Saving Dinner* series. New York: Random House. http://www.savingdinner.com.

Fletcher, Anne. *Weight Loss Confidential: How Teens Lose Weight and Keep It Off.* New York: Houghton Mifflin, 2006.

Food Marketing Institute. "Trends in the United States: Consumer Attitudes and the Supermarket." 2004.

Foreman, Judy. "Eat Fish, Be Happy." *The Boston Globe,* March 8, 2005.

Fujimura, Sara Francis. "Obento American Style." *Tomorrow's Child Magazine,* 2005.

Hassink, Sandra G., M.D., ed. *A Parent's Guide to Childhood Obesity: A Road Map to Health.* American Academy of Pediatrics. 2005.

Kalyn, Wayne. "The Best News in Fitness." *Parade,* April 23, 2006.

Kingsolver, Barbara. *Animal, Vegetable, Miracle: A Year of Food Life.* New York: Harper Collins, 2007.

Kolata, Gina. *Rethinking Thin: The New Science of Weight Loss—and the Myths and Realities of Dieting.* New York: Farrar, Straus and Giroux, 2007.

Koplan, Jeffrey P. Liverman, Catharyn T. and Kraak, Vivica A. *Editors,* Committee on Prevention of Obesity in Children and Youth. Preventing Childhood Obesity: Health in the BalanceWashington DC: National Academies Press, 2004.

Krieger, Ellie. *Small Changes, Big Results: A 12-Week Action Plan to a Better Life.* New York: Random House, 2005.

Liebman, Bonnie, and Jayne Hurley. *Healthy Foods: Your Guide to the Best Basic Foods.* Washington DC: Center for Science in the Public Interest, 2004.

Lindner, Larry. "Forgetting to Enjoy Food May Be Unhealthy." *The Boston Globe,* February 22, 2005.

Lindner, Larry. "More Guidelines Add Up to Less Food." *The Boston Globe,* January 25, 2005.

Linn, Susan. *Consuming Kids: The Hostile Takeover of Childhood.* New York: Anchor Books, 2005.

Ludwig, David. *Ending the Food Fight.* Boston: Houghton Mifflin, 2007.

Madison, Deborah. *Local Flavors.* New York: Broadway Books, 2002.

McRandle, P. W. "The Green Guide: The Smart Green Shopper's Food and Drink Label Choices." http://www.thegreenguide.com.

Meltz, Barbara F. "A Preventive for Smoking and Drinking? Try Dining as a Family." *The Boston Globe,* 2005.

Merrell, Kathy. "Hungry for Organic." *Real Simple,* September 2004.

Micco, Nicci. "The Food Pyramid Is Wrong." *Organic Style,* January/February 2004.

Mishra, Raja. "Study Cites Obesity as Longevity Threat." *The Boston Globe,* March 17, 2005.

Moskin, Julia. "Creamy, Healthier Ice Cream? What's the Catch?" *The New York Times,* July 26, 2006.

Moskowitz, Isa Chandra. *Vegan with a Vengeance.* New York: Marlowe and Company, 2005.

National Cancer Institute Fact Sheets. http://www.cancer.gov/cancertopics/factsheet.

Nearing, Helen. *Simple Food for the Good Life.* New York: Delacorte Press, 1980.

Nestle, Marion. *Food Politics: How the Food Industry Influences Nutrition and Health.* Berkeley, California: University of California Press, 2002.

Nestle, Marion, *What to Eat.* New York: North Point Press, 2006.

National Institutes of Health Office of Dietary Supplements: http://ods.od.nih.gov/index.aspx

Nutrition Action Healthletter. "America's Pressure Cooker." July/August 2005.

Panel on Dietary Reference Intakes for Electrolytes and Water Institute of Medicine. *Water, Potassium, Sodium, Chloride, and Sulfate* Washington, D.C., National Academies Press 2004.

"PETA Vegetarian Starter Kit." Norfolk, Virginia: People for the Ethical Treatment of Animals, 2005.

Physicians Committee for Responsible Medicine Nutrition Panel: Patricia R. Bertron, et al. "Vegetarian Diets: Advantages for Children." http://www.pcrm.org/health/veginfo/vegetarian_kids.html.

Physicians Committee for Responsible Medicine. "School Lunch Report Card 2007." http://www.healthyschoollunches.org/reports/report2007_intro.html.

———. "The Healthy School Lunch Campaign." http://www.healthyschoollunches.org.

Pollan, Michael. *The Omnivore's Dilemma: A Natural History of Four Meals.* New York: Penguin Press, 2006.

Robbins, John. *Diet for a New America.* Tiburon CA: H J Kramer, 1987.

Mary Swartz Rose, PhD, *Feeding the Family,* New York: The Macmillan Company, 1940

Ross, Emma. "Health Benefits, Concern Surface in Study of Farm-Raised Fish." *The Boston Globe,* September 2, 2004.

Satter, Ellyn. *How to Get Your Kid to Eat ... But Not Too Much.* Boulder CO: Bull Publishing, 1987.

Schlosser, Eric. *Fast Food Nation.* New York: Houghton Mifflin, 2001.

Schlosser, Eric, and Charles Wilson. *Chew on This.* New York: Houghton Mifflin, 2006.

Shape Up America! "20 Tips for Getting Your Family on Track." http://www.shapeup.org/fittips/20_tips.php

Sherlock, Marie. *Living Simply with Children.* NY: Three Rivers Press, 2003.

Shoul, Paul. "Lessons in Good Eating." *Harvard School of Public Health Review,* Spring 2006.

Singer, Peter, and Jim Mason. *The Way We Eat: Why Our Food Choices Matter.* NY: Rodale Press, 2006.

Sizer, Frances and Whitney, Eleanor. Nutrition Concepts and Controversies: 8th edition Belmont, CA: Wadsworth/Thomson Learning, 2000.

Slow Food International. http://www.slowfood.com.

Slow Food USA. http://www.slowfoodusa.org.

Smith, Stephen. "Report Finds Soft Drinks Increase Risk of Diabetes." *The Boston Globe,* August 25, 2004.

Squires, Sally **The Omega Principle** Some Fish Fats Protect the Heart. What If They Could Also Treat Your Brain? Washington Post. August 19, 2003; Page HE01

Stein, Rob. "Americans a Little Taller, but Much Heavier Than 40 Years Ago." *The Washington Post,* October 28, 2004.

Thich Nhat Hanh. *For a Future to Be Possible: Commentaries on the Five Wonderful Precepts* (1993) by Thich Nhat Hanh. Bekeley, CA: Parallax Press 1993.

The Wellness Letter. http://www.wellnessletter.com.

U.S. Department of Agriculture. Center for Nutrition Policy and Promotion. http://www.mypyramid.gov.

U.S. Food and Drug Administration. "Advisory: What You Need to Know about Mercury in Fish and Shellfish." March 2004, EPA-823-R-04-005. http://www.cfsan.fda.gov.

———. Center for Food Safety and Applied Nutrition. "How to Understand and Use the Nutrition Facts Label." November 2004. http://www.cfscan.fda.gov.

Walker, Barbara M. *The Little House Cookbook.* New York: Harper and Row Publishers, 1979.

Wansink, Brian. *Mindless Eating: Why We Eat More Than We Think.* New York: Bantam Books, 2006.

"When It Pays to Buy Organic." *Consumer Reports,* February 2006.

Wilder, Laura Ingalls. *Farmer Boy.* New York: Harper and Row Publishers, 1933.

Witty, Helen. *Fancy Pantry.* New York: Workman Publishing, 1986.

World Health Organization. "Global Strategy on Diet, Physical Activity, and Health." May 2004. http://www.who.int/dietphysicalactivity/strategy/eb11344/strategy_english_web.pdf.

Willett, Walter MD. Eat Drink and Be Healthy. New York: Simon & Schuster, 2005.

Yunsheng Ma, MD, PhD, Youfu Li, MD, MPH, David E. Chiriboga, MD, MPH, Barbara C. Olendzki, RD, MPH, James R. Hebert, MSPH, ScD, Wenjun Li, PhD, Katherine Leung, MPH, Andrea R. Hafner, BS and Ira S. Ockene, MD "Association between Carbohydrate Intake and Serum Lipids" published in the Journal of the American College of Nutrition, Vol. 25, No. 2, 155–163 (2006)

978-0-595-46760-0
0-595-46760-1

Printed in the United States
201588BV00001B/226-249/P